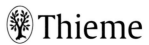

Direct Diagnosis in Radiology

Brain Imaging

Klaus Sartor, MD
Professor of Neuroradiology
Director, Division of Neuroradiology
Department of Neurology
University of Heidelberg Medical Center
Heidelberg, Germany

Stefan Haehnel, MD
Associate Professor of Neuroradiology
Assistant Director, Division of Neuroradiology
Department of Neurology
University of Heidelberg Medical Center
Heidelberg, Germany

Bodo Kress, MD
Clinical Associate Professor of Neuroradiology
Director, Division of Neuroradiology
Department of Radiology and Neuroradiology
Hospital Nordwest
Frankfurt am Main, Germany

336 Illustrations

Thieme
Stuttgart · New York

Library of Congress Cataloging-in-Publication Data is available from the publisher.

This book is an authorized and revised translation of the German edition published and copyrighted 2006 by Georg Thieme Verlag, Stuttgart, Germany. Title of the German edition: Pareto-Reihe Radiologie: Gehirn.

Translator: John Grossman, Schrepkow, Germany

© 2008 Georg Thieme Verlag KG
Rüdigerstrasse 14, 70469 Stuttgart,
Germany
http://www.thieme.de
Thieme New York, 333 Seventh Avenue,
New York, NY 10001, USA
http://www.thieme.com

Cover design: Thieme Publishing Group
Typesetting by Ziegler + Müller,
Kirchentellinsfurt, Germany
Printed by APPL, aprinta Druck,
Wemding, Germany

ISBN 978-3-13-143961-1
(TPS, Rest of World)
ISBN 978-1-58890-570-3
(TPN, The Americas)   1 2 3 4 5 6

Contents

6 Tumors
B. Kress

7 Cysts
B. Kress

8 Meninges
B. Kress

9 Ventricles and Cisterns
S. Haehnel

10 Leukoencephalopathies
S. Haehnel

11 Congenital Malformations
S. Haehnel

12 Artifacts in MRI
S. Haehnel, B. Kress

13 Postoperative Changes
B. Kress, S. Haehnel

ACTH	Adrenocorticotropic hormone	**MALT**	Mucosal associated lymphoid tissue
ADC	Apparent diffusion coefficient	**MELAS**	Mitochondrial myopathy, encephalopathy, lactic acidosis, and stroke-like episodes
ADEM	Acute disseminated encephalomyelitis		
AIDS	Acquired immuno-deficiency syndrome	**MIP**	Maximum intensity projection
ALS	Amyotrophic lateral sclerosis	**MR**	Magnetic resonance
ANA	Antinuclear antibody	**MRA**	Magnetic resonance angiography
ANCA	Antineutrophil cyto-plasmic antibodies	**MRI**	Magnetic resonance imaging
AVM	Arteriovenous malformation	**MRS**	Magnetic resonance spectroscopy
C	Cervical vertebra	**MS**	Multiple sclerosis
CADASIL	Cerebral autosomal domi-nant arteriopathy with subcortical infarcts and leukoencephalopathy	**MT**	Magnetization transfer
		PDGF	Platelet derived growth factor
		PET	Positron emission tomography
CBF	Cerebral blood flow		
CNS	Central nervous system	**PML**	Progressive multifocal leukoencephalopathy
CSF	Cerebrospinal fluid		
CT	Computed tomography, computed tomogram	**PVL**	Periventricular leukomalacia
CTA	CT angiography	**rCBF**	Regional cerebral blood flow
DNT	Dysembryoplastic neuroepithelial tumor	**rMTT**	Relative mean transit time
DSA	Digital subtraction angiography	**ROI**	Region of interest
		rrCBV	Relative regional cerebral blood volume
EGFR	Epidermal growth factor receptor		
		SAH	Subarachnoid hemorrhage
F	Female	**SDH**	Subdural hematoma
FLAIR	Fluid-attenuated inversion recovery	**SPECT**	Single-photon emission computed tomography
HIV	Human immunodeficiency virus	**STH**	Somatotropic hormone
		TE	echo time
HSV	Herpes simplex virus	**TOF**	Time of flight
HU	Hounsfield unit	**TRUE FISP**	True fast imaging with steady state precession
IR	Inversion recovery		
IV	Intravenous	**V2**	Maxillary nerve
M	Male	**V3**	Mandibular nerve

Definition

▶ **Epidemiology**
  The most common type of bleeding in craniocerebral trauma.
▶ **Etiology, pathophysiology, pathogenesis**
  Traumatic intra-axial bleeding • Injury to cerebral parenchyma • May occur in combination with other forms of hematoma (subdural, subarachnoid, intracerebral) in up to 20% of all cases • Localization: frontobasal, occipital, parietal.

Imaging Signs

▶ **Modality of choice**
  CT.
▶ **CT findings**
  Hypodense in the acute stage, later hyperdense with a hypodense halo (perifocal edema) • Size: a few millimeters to several centimeters • Bleeding at point of impact and contrecoup bleeding are present, whereby the size of the contrecoup hemorrhage can be larger than that at the point of impact • There may be a mass effect depending on the size of the hemorrhage and the extent of the edema:
  – Cerebral swelling with reduced definition of the cortex.
  – Midline displacement.
  – Compression of ventricular system with obstructed flow of CSF.
  – Compression of the cisterna ambiens.
▶ **MRI findings**
  Not indicated in diagnosing acute cases • High sensitivity for older hemorrhages (subacute to chronic) • Hypointense susceptibility artifact on T2*-weighted images • Signal intensity on T1- and T2-weighted images corresponds to that of the bleeding in the respective stage of the hemoglobin breakdown process (p. 101).

Clinical Aspects

▶ **Typical presentation**
  Often unspecific, depending on the extent of bleeding • Headache • Vomiting • Nausea • Vertigo • Alertness is impaired, occasionally to point of loss of consciousness • Hemiparesis • Oculomotor impairment.
▶ **Treatment options**
  Surgical treatment is rarely indicated • Observation and control of edema are usually sufficient • Bleeding into the ventricular system may require drainage of cerebrospinal fluid.
▶ **Course and prognosis**
  This depends on the extent of the bleeding.
▶ **What does the clinician want to know?**
  Localization • Extent • Mass effect • Impingement • Rupture into the ventricular system • Obstructed flow of CSF.

Fig. 1.1 Hemorrhagic contusion in the superior frontal gyrus, 24 hours old. Axial CT.

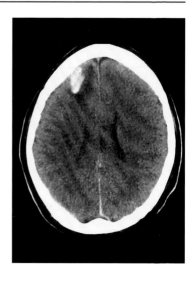

Differential Diagnosis

The various forms of bleeding can occur in combination, rendering a differential diagnosis difficult.

Hemorrhagic infarction	– Significant perifocal edema usually present initially
	– Significantly reduced ADC
Venous infarction	– Atypical location of hemorrhage (e.g. temporooccipital)
	– No history of trauma
	– Significant surrounding edema usually present initially
Congophilic hemorrhage	– Usually multifocal hemorrhages (T2*-weighted MR image)
	– Additional signs suggestive of microangiopathy

Tips and Pitfalls

CT too early: Cerebral contusion may only be detectable after several hours. Therefore, a follow-up examination of intubated patients is indicated within six hours •
Conscious patients should undergo a follow-up examination the following day.

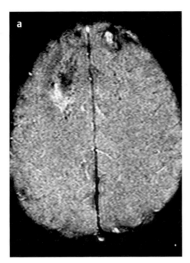
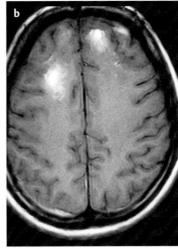

Fig. 1.2 a, b Bifrontal hemorrhagic contusion 3–4 days old. Axial T2*-weighted MR image (**a**) and axial T1-weighted MR image (**b**). Loss of signal due to susceptibility artifact on T2*-weighted images (**a**). Hyperintense signal (methemoglobin) on the T1-weighted image (**b**).

Selected References

Parizel P et al. Intracranial hemorrhage: Principles of CT and MRI interpretation. Europ Radiol 2001; 11 (9): 1770–1783

Struffert T et al. Schädel- und Hirntrauma. Radiologe 2003; 43: 861–877

Wiesmann M et al. Bildgebende Diagnostik akuter Schädel-Hirn-Verletzungen. Radiologe 1998; 38: 645–658

Definition

▸ **Etiology, pathophysiology, pathogenesis**
Stretched or torn nerve fibers ● Loss of neurons ● Petechial hemorrhage where perineural vessels are involved ● Only about 20% of the lesions are hemorrhagic ● Only half of the cases are posttraumatic; drug use is the next most common cause (recurrent hypoxia) ● Disorder is most commonly supratentorial, in order of decreasing incidence: frontotemporal white matter—corpus callosum—brainstem.

Imaging Signs

▸ **Modality of choice**
MRI.
▸ **CT findings**
Findings are often unimpressive in the acute phase ● Follow-up examinations demonstrate hemorrhages measuring a few millimeters at the corticomedullary junction ● Edema is absent ● Lesions in the corpus callosum and brainstem are difficult to detect ● Nonhemorrhagic shear injuries cannot be diagnosed ● Atrophy is a late sign of a shear injury.
▸ **MRI findings**
T2*-weighted images will show a hemosiderin effect from hemorrhagic shear injuries ● The apparent diffusion coefficient (ADC) is reduced ● Usually at the corticomedullary junction ● Linear or oval shaped ● No surrounding edema ● Often demonstrated only by histologic findings as many injuries are not detectable on MR images, especially nonhemorrhagic injuries.

Clinical Aspects

▸ **Typical presentation**
The critical clinical condition is inconsistent with the "harmless" CT findings ● Consciousness is severely impaired ● Decerebrate rigidity ● Convulsions ● Intubation indicated.
▸ **Treatment options**
No specific therapy is available ● Control of edema ● Management of acute complications.
▸ **Course and prognosis**
Poor prognosis ● Protracted convalescence ● Atrophy indicative of loss of neurons.
▸ **What does the clinician want to know?**
Differentiate from a "normal" cerebral contusion ● Course.

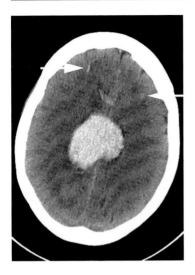

Fig. 1.3 Diffuse axonal injury. Axial CT. Streaklike hemorrhages in the white matter (arrows). Hemorrhage in the corpus callosum and cingulate gyrus.

Differential Diagnosis

Contusion hemorrhage	– Perifocal edema – Typically frontobasal and also occipital
Subarachnoid hemorrhage	– Blood in the sulci
Calcifications	– Do not show dynamic development on follow-up studies
Microangiopathy	– Periventricular location – Located deep in white matter – Does not show dynamic development on follow-up studies at short intervals

Tips and Pitfalls

Failing to consider diffuse axonal injury • An MRI study need not be obtained in the early phase, i.e., within the first seven days. Only in this phase is it possible to demonstrate the injury on the basis of the reduced apparent diffusion.

Trauma

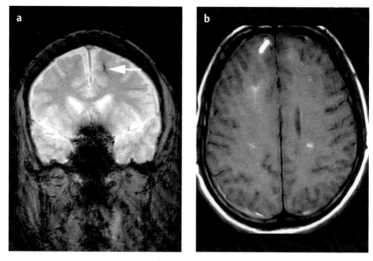

Fig. 1.4a, b Coronal T2*-weighted (**a**) and axial T1-weighted MR images (**b**). Susceptibility artifact on the T2*-weighted image (**a**). After a few days the hemorrhages are also
recognizable on the T1-weighted images by their hyperintense signal (**b**).

Selected References

Chan J et al. Diffuse axonal injury: detection of changes in anisotropy of water diffusion by
diffusion-weighted imaging. Neuroradiology 2003; 45: 34–38

Niess C et al. Incidence of axonal injury in human brain tissue. Acta Neuropathol 2002;
104: 79–84

Struffert T et al. Schädel- und Hirntrauma. Radiologe 2003; 43: 861–877

Definition

▶ **Epidemiology**
Incidence: 10–20% of all patients with craniocerebral trauma.

▶ **Etiology, pathophysiology, pathogenesis**
Acute or chronic accumulation of blood between the dura mater and arachnoid •
Usually venous bleeding • Acute subdural hematomas are an absolute emergency indication • Combinations with other forms of hematoma (subdural, subarachnoid, intracerebral) may occur in up to 20% of all cases • In 95% of all cases,
the lesion is supratentorial (especially frontoparietal) • Bilateral hematoma is
present in 15% of all cases.

Imaging Signs

▶ **Modality of choice**
CT.

▶ **Findings on plain skull radiography**
Obsolete study as it can only demonstrate a fracture, but not a cerebral hemorrhage.

▶ **CT findings**
Acute subdural hematoma: Hyperdense crescent-shaped hemorrhage along the
brain (early acute components can appear hypodense) • Not bounded by sutures • Significant mass effect: midline displacement (may be absent in bilateral
hematomas) • Obstructed flow of CSF, blockage of the interventricular foramen
of Monro • Reduced demarcation between gray and white matter • Cisterna ambiens obliterated • In infratentorial hematomas the cerebellar tonsils are displaced into the foramen magnum • The medial temporal lobe may become impinged in the tentorial notch • Usually there is no visible fracture • Frequently
occurs in combination with intra-axial bleeding • Postoperative contralateral rebleeding may occur in response to removal of the tamponade.
Chronic subdural hematoma: Isodense or hypodense extra-axial collection of
blood in a crescent along the brain • Lesion crosses suture lines • With isointense hematomas, the midline displacement is often the only detectable sign
of a hematoma (selecting a wider CT window than normal is helpful) • The contrast enhancement of the cerebral vessels after IV administration of contrast
agent aids in differentiating the hematoma from brain tissue • Significant mass
effect • Usually there is no fracture.

▶ **MRI findings**
MRI is not indicated in an acute subdural hematoma • In a chronic subdural
hematoma, MRI can be used to estimate the age of the lesion (signal intensity
of the hemoglobin breakdown products is helpful in a medical opinion, p. 101).

Fig. 1.5 Acute hemorrhage in a chronic subdural hematoma. Axial CT. Acute blood with mass effect is visualized next to chronic hypodense blood (*). In contrast to acute epidural hematoma, the subdural hematoma is concave and not limited by cranial sutures.

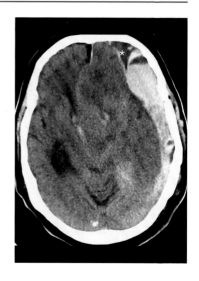

Clinical Aspects

▶ **Typical presentation**

Acute subdural hematoma: Absolute emergency indication ● Clinical findings are similar to epidural hematoma ● Nausea, vomiting, headache, unconsciousness ● The patient's condition can dramatically worsen very rapidly ● Anisocoria or suddenly fixed pupils are an alarm signal but a late sign ● Patients are often intubated.

Chronic subdural hematoma: Clinical signs are relatively mild compared with CT findings ● Headache, nausea, vomiting, vertigo ● Slowed reactions, listlessness, signs of dementia ● Hemiparesis symptoms occur rarely ● Follow-up examination is indicated within 6–24 hours of initial examination, depending on clinical findings.

▶ **Treatment options**

Craniotomy ● Immediately indicated in subdural hematoma; treatment the next day may be acceptable in chronic hematoma.

▶ **Course and prognosis**

Chronic subdural hematomas may recur ● Prognosis is usually poor due to concomitant administration of drugs such as acetylsalicylic acid and clopidogrel.

▶ **What does the clinician want to know?**

Extent ● Midline displacement ● Size of basal cisterns ● Obstructed flow of CSF.

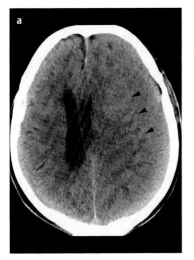 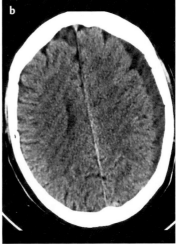

Fig. 1.6 a, b Chronological development of a chronic subdural hematoma in CT images. Two to three weeks after the hemorrhage, the hematoma exhibits densities approximately equal to that of brain tissue (**a**). This makes it difficult to delineate hematoma from brain tissue (arrowheads). During the further clinical course, the density of the hematoma decreases to values similar to CSF (**b**).

Differential Diagnosis

Epidural hematoma	– Convex, crescentic
	– Does not cross suture line
Subarachnoid hematoma	– Blood is visible in the sulci
	– No midline displacement
Intracerebral hematoma	– Bleeding into cerebral parenchyma
Subdural abscess	– Septic clinical syndrome
	– Comorbidities usually present
	– Hypodense or isodense to brain tissue, significant contrast enhancement
	– No history of recent trauma

Tips and Pitfalls

Failing to detect bilateral isodense chronic subdural hematomas.

Fig. 1.7   Acute subdural hematoma in the posterior longitudinal fissure and in a frontal location. Axial CT.

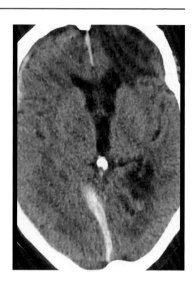

Selected References

Maxeiner H. Entstehungsbedingungen, Quellen und Typologie von tödlichen Subdural-blutungen. Rechtsmedizin 1998; 9 (1): 14–20

Struffert T et al. Schädel- und Hirntrauma. Radiologe 2003; 43: 861–877

Wiesmann M et al. Bildgebende Diagnostik akuter Schädel-Hirn-Verletzungen. Radiologe 1998; 38: 645– 658

Definition

▶ **Epidemiology**
Frequency: 1–5% of all patients with craniocerebral trauma ● In 5% of these cases bilaterally (occasionally only after surgical decompression of one side).

▶ **Etiology, pathophysiology, pathogenesis**
Acute, usually traumatic bleeding between the inner table and dura mater ● Usually the result of arterial injury (middle meningeal artery in 85% of all cases) ● Venous bleeding occurs in 15% of all cases (diploic veins, dural venous sinus, especially in infratentorial hematomas) ● May occur in combination with other forms of hematoma (subdural, subarachnoid, intracerebral) in up to 20% of all cases ● Localization: usually temporoparietal.

Imaging Signs

▶ **Modality of choice**
CT.

▶ **Findings on plain skull radiography**
Obsolete study as the film can only demonstrate a fracture, but not the extent of bleeding ● Obtaining a plain skull film merely delays relevant diagnostic studies.

▶ **CT findings**
Semiconvex shape ● Hyperdense ● Acute, uncoagulated blood components can also be hypodense ● The hematoma cannot cross suture lines as the dura mater is firmly attached to the bone along the boundaries of the calvaria ● Significant mass effect: midline displacement ● Reduced demarcation between gray and white matter ● Obstructed flow of CSF (blockage of the interventricular foramen of Monro) ● Cisterna ambiens narrowed (the medial temporal lobe may become impinged in the tentorial notch) ● The hematoma can rapidly expand ● Usually there is a displaced calvarial fracture ● Postoperative contralateral rebleeding (epidural or intracerebral) may occur in response to removal of the tamponade.

▶ **MRI findings**
Not indicated because of the long time required to organize and perform the examination.

Clinical Aspects

▶ **Typical presentation**
Absolute emergency that can rapidly become life threatening ● Nausea, vomiting, headache, unconsciousness ● The patient's condition can dramatically worsen very rapidly ● Anisocoria or suddenly fixed pupils are an alarm signal but a late sign ● Patients are often intubated.

▶ **Treatment options**
Surgery is usually indicated ● Unconscious patients with an epidural hematoma not requiring surgery should have a follow-up CT within six hours ● Conscious patients who can undergo neurologic evaluation may have a follow-up CT the

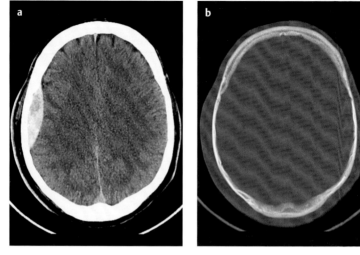

Fig. 1.8 a, b Epidural hematoma. Axial CT. Convex, hyperdense mass close to the calvaria. The sutures are a natural barrier for epidural hematomas because here the dura mater is firmly attached to the calvaria (**a**). Epidural hematomas typically occur in the setting of a fracture (**b**).

next day ● Patients with an epidural hematoma not requiring surgery must remain under observation (ideally in the intensive care unit).
▶ **Course and prognosis**
With early craniotomy, the prognosis is good; otherwise mortality is high.
▶ **What does the clinician want to know?**
Extent ● Midline displacement ● Obstructed flow of CSF.

Differential Diagnosis

Subdural hematoma	– Crosses suture line
	– Significant mass effect even with minimal thickness
	– Symptoms milder, especially in chronic hematomas
	– Often no visible fracture
Subarachnoid hematoma	– Blood visible deep in the sulci
	– No midline displacement
Intracerebral hematoma	– Bleeding into cerebral parenchyma
Epidural abscess	– Septic clinical syndrome
	– Comorbidities usually present
	– Hypodense or isodense to brain tissue
	– No history of recent trauma

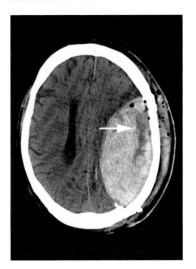

Fig. 1.9 Postoperative epidural bleeding. Axial CT. Acute epidural hematomas can also contain hypodense components (arrow). This is acute blood that has not yet coagulated. The air inclusions are residues of the operation.

Tips and Pitfalls

No follow-up examination • No observation on the ward • Failing to detect temporal polar epidural hematoma.

Selected References

Struffert T et al. Schädel- und Hirntrauma. Radiologe 2003; 43: 861–877
Wiesmann M et al. Bildgebende Diagnostik akuter Schädel-Hirn Verletzungen. Radiologe 1998; 38: 645–658

Definition

▶ **Etiology, pathophysiology, pathogenesis**
Bleeding into the subarachnoid space secondary to trauma • Rupture of veins or arteries • May occur in combination with hematomas at other sites (subdural, subarachnoid, intracerebral) in up to 20% of all cases • Typical localization: parietal.

Imaging Signs

▶ **Modality of choice**
CT.

▶ **Findings on plain skull radiography**
Obsolete study as the film can only demonstrate a fracture, but not the extent of bleeding.

▶ **CT findings**
Streaks in the sulci isodense to blood • Typical localization: parietal • No midline displacement • No evidence of aneurysm on arterial CT angiography • Flow of CSF may be obstructed.

▶ **MRI findings**
Prepontine hemorrhages are best visualized on proton density-weighted images (hyperintense signal in hypointense CSF) • Subarachnoid hemorrhages in the cerebral hemispheres are best visualized on FLAIR images (hyperintense signal of the sulci) • Chronic subarachnoid hemorrhages appear on T2*-weighted images as a hypointense coating over the surface of the brain (siderosis, p. 244).

Clinical Aspects

▶ **Typical presentation**
Craniocerebral trauma dominates the clinical picture • An isolated traumatic subarachnoid hemorrhage is a rare finding • Headache, nausea, vomiting • Vertigo • Consciousness is impaired, occasionally to point of loss of consciousness • Obstructed flow of CSF.

▶ **Treatment options**
Management of complications.

▶ **Course and prognosis**
This depends on the severity of the craniocerebral trauma.

▶ **What does the clinician want to know?**
Differentiate from a subarachnoid hemorrhage due to a ruptured aneurysm • Obstructed flow of CSF.

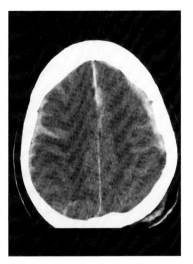

Fig. 1.10 Traumatic subarachnoid hemorrhage. Axial CT. Hyperdense frontoparietal subarachnoid space. Adjacent to this is a subdural hematoma on the left side.

Differential Diagnosis

The sensitivity of CT for demonstrating a subarachnoid hemorrhage is at most 90%; this means a normal CT does not exclude a subarachnoid hemorrhage • MRI has the same sensitivity as lumbar puncture.

Aneurysmal hemorrhage	– In the basal cisterns or prepontine region
	– Proven aneurysm is diagnostic
	– Differential diagnosis can be difficult, especially with uncertain trauma; such cases require identical diagnostic procedures as aneurysmal hemorrhage (CTA, DSA)

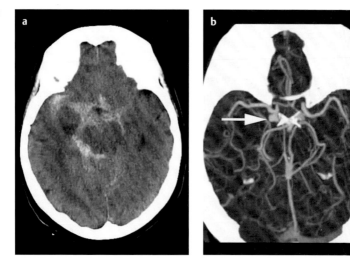

Fig. 1.11 a, b Aneurysmal subarachnoid hemorrhage. Axial CT (**a**) and CTA (**b**). In contrast to traumatic subarachnoid hemorrhage, the greater portion of the blood in an aneurysmal hemorrhage is in the basal cisterns (**a**). Aneurysm demonstrated on arterial CTA (**b**, arrow).

Tips and Pitfalls
• •

Misinterpreting a ruptured aneurysm as a traumatic subarachnoid hemorrhage •
When in doubt, at least perform CT angiography.

Selected References
Grunwald I et al. Klinik, Diagnostik und Therapie der Subarachnoidalblutung. Radiologe 2002; 42: 860–870
Struffert T et al. Schädel- und Hirntrauma. Radiologe 2003; 43: 861–877
Wiesmann M et al. Nachweis der akuten Subarachnoidalblutung. FLAIR und Protonen-dichte-gewichtete MRT-Sequenzen bei 1,5 Tesla. Radiologe 1999; 39: 860–865

Definition

▶ **Epidemiology**
Frequency: Occurs in 20% of all severe craniocerebral trauma cases ● Frequently accompanies tumors and infarctions as well.

▶ **Etiology, pathophysiology, pathogenesis**
Inclusion of fluid in the brain parenchyma (vasogenic, cytotoxic) ● Impaired cerebral vascular autoregulation ● Hypoxia ● The swelling can briefly occur secondary to trauma, but usually only a day or two later.

Imaging Signs

▶ **Modality of choice**
CT or MRI.

▶ **CT findings**
Loss of demarcation between gray and white matter ● Increase in the volume of brain parenchyma, decrease in the volume of the subarachnoid space and cisterns ● White matter is hypodense ● Mass effect is present, which may include herniation ● Intact portions of the brain are visualized adjacent to edematous portions (for example, "white cerebellum sign").

▶ **MRI findings**
Loss of demarcation between gray and white matter ● On T1-weighted inversion recovery images, the otherwise typical contrast between the hypointense gray matter and hyperintense white matter is no longer discernible ● The apparent diffusion coefficient (ADC) is reduced in cytotoxic cerebral edema and increased in vasogenic and interstitial cerebral edema ● Obstructed flow of CSF.

Clinical Aspects

▶ **Typical presentation**
Life-threatening clinical syndrome ● Patients usually require intubation and assisted respiration.

▶ **Treatment options**
Control of edema: mannitol, appropriate physical steps ● Hemicraniotomy where indicated.

▶ **Course and prognosis**
Up to 50% mortality.

▶ **What does the clinician want to know?**
Mass effect (extent of midline displacement in millimeters, impingement signs, obstructed flow of CSF, infarctions) ● Signs of brain death.

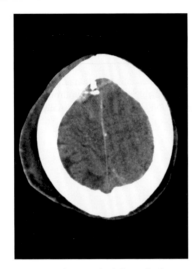

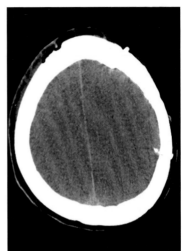

Fig. 1.12 Edema in the left cerebral hemisphere. Axial CT. Compared with the right side, the left sulci are less clearly delineated and the demarcation between gray and white matter is reduced.

Fig. 1.13 Hypoxia. Axial CT. Absence of demarcation between gray and white matter. The sulci are no longer delineated, indicating irreversible damage to the cerebral parenchyma.

Differential Diagnosis

Brain not yet fully myelinized

– Normal demarcation between gray and white matter, although no sulci can be delineated
– No asymmetry between the hemispheres

Tips and Pitfalls

Failing to identify herniation (p. 19).

Selected References

Karantanas A et al. Contribution of MRI and MR angiography in early diagnosis of brain death. Europ Radiol 2002; 12 (11): 2710–2716

Struffert T et al. Schädel- und Hirntrauma. Teil 2: Intraaxiale Verletzungen, sekundäre Verletzungen. Radiologe 2003; 43: 1001–1016

Definition

▶ **Etiology, pathophysiology, pathogenesis**
The falx and tentorium divide the intracranial space into two supratentorial spaces and an infratentorial space ● A hemorrhage or cerebral edema forces brain tissue into an adjacent compartment: subfalcial herniation (midline displacement), transtentorial or tonsilar herniation ● Herniation syndromes lead to ischemic lesions and obstructed flow of CSF, which may eventually cause death if they persist.

Imaging Signs

▶ **Modality of choice**
CT.
▶ **CT findings**
CT systems with multiple detectors allow multiplanar reconstructions that visualize the displacement of brain tissue.
Subfalcial herniation: Most common herniation syndrome ● The septum pellucidum is displaced to the contralateral side (semiconvex course) ● There is a risk of obstructed flow of CSF due to blockage of the interventricular foramen of Monro (the width of the temporal horns is a sensitive sign of this).
Transtentorial herniation: Displacement of portions of the midbrain inferiorly through the tentorium ● Narrowing or complete occlusion (obliteration) of the cisterna ambiens ● Usually with midline displacement ● Obstructed flow of CSF due to compression of the sylvian aqueduct.
Tonsilar herniation: Infratentorial mass effect ● Displacement of the cerebellar tonsils inferiorly through the foramen magnum ● Obliteration of the prepontine cistern ● The perimedullar halo of CSF is no longer present in the foramen magnum ● Obstructed flow of CSF due to compression of the sylvian aqueduct and the fourth ventricle.
▶ **MRI findings**
This modality is the second choice due to the time it requires ● Multiplanar imaging can visualize the herniation syndrome in all planes ● Secondary sequelae that can be visualized include: microhemorrhages (T2*-weighted images), cranial nerve lesions (T1-weighted gradient echo sequences after injection of contrast agent), hypoxic brain damage (diffusion-weighted images).

Clinical Aspects

▶ **Typical presentation**
Severely ill patient, usually intubated and requiring assisted respiration ● Life-threatening situation, especially where there is impingement in the tentorial notch and foramen magnum ● Pupillomotor dysfunction ● Brainstem syndrome with loss of corneal reflex, altered respiration, and cardiovascular dysfunction ● Obstructed flow of CSF.

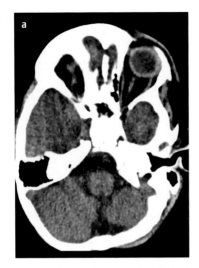 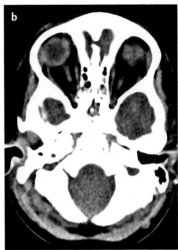

Fig. 1.14 a, b Development of cerebral edema in craniocerebral trauma. Axial CT. At admission to the hospital (**a**) the prepontine cistern is still completely intact. Two days after trauma (**b**) there is significant infratentorial swelling. The intracranial portion of the cisterna magna at the foramen magnum is no longer visible. The cerebellar tonsils are displaced into the foramen magnum (inferior impingement).

▶ **Treatment options**
Control of edema, for example with mannitol ● Appropriate physical steps ● Decompression craniotomy.

▶ **Course and prognosis**
Life-threatening situation with poor prognosis.

▶ **What does the clinician want to know?**
Are the basal cisterns still demarcated? ● Obstructed flow of CSF? ● Signs of brain death?

Differential Diagnosis
....

Chiari malformation	– Cerebellar tonsils extend into the foramen magnum but secondary signs are absent (prepontine space not narrowed)
Asymmetrically positioned patient	– Septum pellucidum in the center – No sequelae of trauma

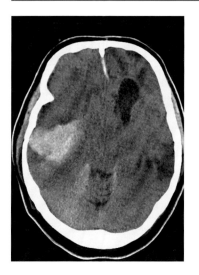

Fig. 1.15 Axial CT. Significant midline shift with blockage of the foramen of Monro due to the right temporal hemorrhage (widening of the left lateral ventricle). Narrowing of the perimesencephalic cisterns (transtentorial herniation).

Tips and Pitfalls

Misinterpreting a Chiari malformation as impingement • Failing to note the width of the basal cisterns.

Selected References

Struffert T et al. Schädel- und Hirntrauma. Teil 2: Intraxiale Verletzungen, sekundäre Verletzungen. Radiologe 2003; 43: 861–877

Trauma

Definition

▶ **Epidemiology**
Frequency: Occurs in approximately 3% of all patients with craniocerebral trauma • Intracranial injury is present in 90% of all patients with skull fracture.

▶ **Etiology, pathophysiology, pathogenesis**
Traumatic discontinuity of the calvaria or facial portion of the skull • Discontinuity of the inner and outer tables.

Imaging Signs

▶ **Modality of choice**
CT.

▶ **Plain skull radiography**
Such studies are obsolete as they cannot exclude intracranial injury • Guidelines of the German Society of Neuropediatrics specify CT as the modality of choice for primary diagnosis of craniocerebral trauma where available • Conventional radiographs are only helpful in isolated facial trauma (submentobregmatic "jug handle" view in a fracture of the zygomatic arch, occipitomental/occipitofrontal nasal sinus views in a midfacial fracture) • Look for indirect fracture signs (fluid levels, air).

▶ **CT findings**
Should be recalculated in the bone algorithm and documented in the bone window, for example, w 400 c 1500 • Discontinuity of the calvaria traceable through several slices • Midfacial fractures require multiplanar reconstructions, for example, coronal in an orbital floor fracture and sagittal in a temporomandibular joint fracture • Fluid in the petrous bone or nasal sinuses is an indirect fracture sign in patients with craniocerebral trauma • Intracranial air is a sign of an open fracture of the frontal or temporal base • CSF leaks are difficult to diagnose; sometimes this is possible only with intrathecal contrast (CT with the patient prone).

▶ **MRI findings**
In injuries to the atlantoaxial junction • Fat-saturated T2-weighted images show a hyperintense bone marrow edema.

Clinical Aspects

▶ **Typical presentation**
Retrograde amnesia • Headache • Vomiting, nausea • Vertigo • Cranial CT is absolutely indicated in a unconscious patient with multiple trauma or in patients taking anticoagulants • Clinically asymptomatic patients do not require imaging studies (and especially not a plain skull radiograph).

▶ **Treatment options**
Isolated nondisplaced skull fractures without associated intracranial bleeding are not treated • Displaced fractures can be an indication for surgery.

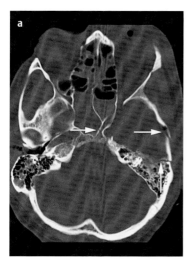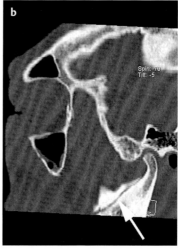

Fig. 1.16 a, b   Multiple skull base fractures (arrows; **a**) in the petrous bone, temporal bone, wall of the sphenoidal sinus, and muscular process of the mandible (arrow; **b**). High-resolution axial CT (**a**) and oblique sagittal reconstruction (**b**).

▶ **Course and prognosis**
The prognosis for nondisplaced fractures without associated intracranial bleeding is good.

▶ **What does the clinician want to know?**
Associated intracranial injury • Displacement of bone fragments.

Differential Diagnosis

Chronic fracture	– Rounded edges in contrast to acute fracture
	– No corresponding soft-tissue swelling
Suture	– Not easy to differentiate from a fracture, especially in children
	– Margin sclerosed
	– Usually symmetrical
	– At typical locations: lambdoid suture, temporo-zygomatic suture, sagittal suture, coronal suture
Ruptured suture	– Asymmetrically widened suture
	– Usually with associated intracranial injury

Fig. 1.17 Fracture of the floor and the roof of the left side orbit. High-resolution axial CT, three-dimensional reconstruction. The extent of fracture displacement is visualized in three dimensions to facilitate preoperative planning.

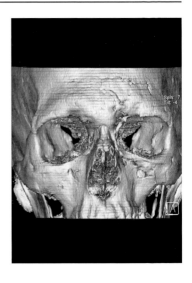

Anomalies	– Various anomalies, especially at the skull base, for example bone defect in the floor of the orbit, lamina papyracea, occipital squama
	– No accompanying symptoms, no hematoma, no soft-tissue swelling
	– Clinical findings do not suggest injury

Tips and Pitfalls

Taking no further action after failing to detect a skull fracture on a plain skull radiograph • Failing to recommend further observation on the ward after diagnosing a skull fracture diagnosed on CT • Failing to diagnose an axially coursing calvarial fracture on CT (scout view is helpful).

Selected References

Leitlinien der Gesellschaft für Neuropädiatrie (gemeinsam mit der Deutschen Gesellschaft für Neurotraumatologie und Klinische Neuropsychologie DGNKN, dem Executive Committee der Euroacademia Multidisciplinaria Neurotraumatologica EMN). Leitlinien der Unfallchirurgie der AWMF: Leitlinie Polytrauma

Struffert T et al. Schädel- und Hirntrauma. Radiologe 2003; 43: 861–877

Wiesmann M et al. Bildgebende Diagnostik akuter Schädel-Hirn-Verletzungen. Radiologe 1998; 38: 645–658

Definition

▶ **Epidemiology**
Morbidity in Central Europe: 50:100 000 ● M:F = 1:2.

▶ **Etiology, pathophysiology, pathogenesis**
Chronic inflammatory demyelinating disorder of the brain and spinal cord ● Inflammation is multifocal (plaques) and diffuse with myelin destruction ● Etiology is unknown.

Imaging Signs

▶ **Modality of choice**
MRI.

▶ **CT findings**
Normal where involvement is slight ● With severe involvement, plaques appear as hypodensities that occasionally enhance with contrast.

▶ **MRI findings**
Focal hyperintensities in the periventricular white matter, corpus callosum ("Dawson's fingers" phenomenon), brainstem or midbrain, and cerebellum on T2-weighted, proton density-weighted, and FLAIR images ● There is a nodular or ring-shaped pattern of enhancement, depending on activity ● IV contrast is not recommended after systemic administration of steroids as even active plaques will usually not enhance in this case ● Active enhancing lesions with an edematous halo will be visualized adjacent to chronic lesions without edema or enhancement ● Adjacent hypointense and isointense foci are visualized on T1-weighted images ● Plaques on non-contrast-enhanced T1-weighted images are hypointense or isointense to normal white matter: Demyelination is more severe in T1-weighted hypointense plaques ("black holes") than in isointense plaques.

Spatial dissemination: At least three of the following four criteria (McDonald criteria) must be fulfilled for radiologic diagnosis:

1. At least one lesion with contrast enhancement or, failing that, nine hyperintense lesions on T2-weighted or FLAIR images.
2. At least one infratentorial lesion.
3. At least one subcortical lesion.
4. At least three periventricular lesions and proven dissemination over time.

A spinal cord lesion is equivalent to an infratentorial lesion.

Dissemination over time:

1. An enhancing lesion demonstrated at least three months after onset of the initial clinical event unless the location of the lesion corresponds with initial symptoms, or
2. A new lesion demonstrated at that time on T2-weighted images in comparison with a reference study obtained at least 30 days before onset of the initial clinical event.

Apparent diffusion coefficient (ADC) in acute plaques is nearly always higher than in chronic plaques, although in rare cases it is reduced.

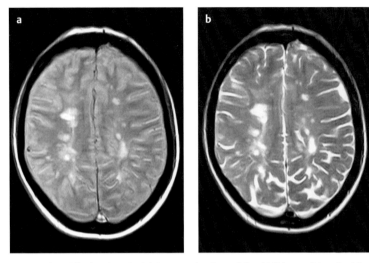

Fig. 2.1a, b Multiple sclerosis. Axial proton density-weighted MR image (**a**) and axial T2-weighted MR image (**b**). Focal hyperintensities in the periventricular white matter.

Clinical Aspects

▶ **Typical presentation**
Onset is typically between the ages of 20 and 40 years ● Initial retrobulbar optic neuritis occurs in approximately 25% of all patients ● Additional initial symptoms include bilateral internuclear ophthalmoplegia, transient cranial nerve palsy or sensory deficits in the area supplied by the trigeminal nerve, and weakness or numbness in the arms and legs.

▶ **Treatment options**
Glucocorticoids in acute episodes ● Episode prophylaxis includes immunotherapy agents (interferons, 1a and 1b immunglobulins, glatiramer acetate) or cytostatic agents (mitoxantrone, cyclophosphamide).

▶ **Course and prognosis**
The clinical course is initially episodic in nearly 80% of all patients ● Secondary chronic progression occurs in about half the patients within 10 years.

▶ **What does the clinician want to know?**
Differentiate from other white matter lesions (such as microangiopathy) ● Differentiate from acute disseminated encephalomyelitis (p. 30).

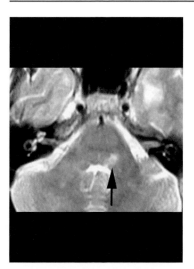

Fig. 2.2 Multiple sclerosis. Axial T2-weighted MR image. Focal hyperintensities in the brainstem (arrow).

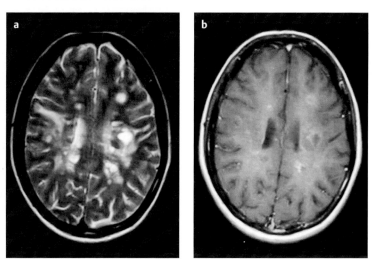

Fig. 2.3 a, b Multiple sclerosis. Axial T2-weighted MR image (**a**) and axial T1-weighted MR image after contrast administration (**b**). Focal hyperintensities in the periventricular white matter (**a**). Nodular or ring enhancement depending on activity (**b**).

Inflammation

Fig. 2.4 Multiple sclerosis. Sagittal T2-weighted MR image. Focal hyperintensities on the inferior aspect of the corpus callosum, "Dawson's fingers" phenomenon.

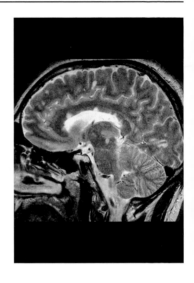

Differential Diagnosis

Embolic or hemodynamic ischemia	– Pattern of distribution corresponds to area supplied by one or more vessels
	– In acute stage ADC invariably reduced
Cerebral vasculitis	– Periventricular white matter and corpus callosum usually not involved
	– Gray matter often involved
CADASIL	– Subcortical infarctions, most often in the frontal and temporal regions (beginning in the temporopolar region) and in the inner capsule
	– Positive family history
	– DNA analysis (gene defect on chromosome 19q12 from mutation of the notch 3 gene)
Brain metastases and other neoplasms	– All of these lesions enhance and exhibit perifocal edema
Postinfectious demyelination as in ADEM	– All lesions in the same stage, i.e., active enhancing lesions with edematous halo, are not seen together with chronic lesions without edema or enhancement.
	– Hypointense and isointense lesions are not seen together on T1-weighted MR images as in multiple sclerosis

Tips and Pitfalls

Administering IV contrast despite glucocorticoid therapy ● Not obtaining sagittal T2-weighted or FLAIR images ● Missing plaques close to the ventricles ● Misinterpreting microangiopathy as multiple sclerosis.

Selected References

Antel J. Multiple sclerosis – emerging concepts of disease pathogenesis. J Neuroimmunol 1999; 98 (1): 45–48

Harting I et al. Bildgebung, Diagnosekriterien und Differenzialdiagnose der Multiplen Sklerose. Röfo Fortschr Geb Röntgenstr Neuen Bildgeb Verfahr 2003; 175 (5): 613–622

McDonald WI et al. Recommended diagnostic criteria for multiple sclerosis: guidelines from the International Panel on the diagnosis of multiple sclerosis. Ann Neurol 2001; 50 (1): 121–127

Definition

▶ **Epidemiology**
Frequency: 1–2:100 000 • *Peak age:* 3–5 years • The disorder can manifest itself at any age.

▶ **Etiology, pathophysiology, pathogenesis**
Histopathology resembles multiple sclerosis, with acute demyelinating inflammation of the brain and spinal cord • In contrast to MS, the course is monophasic • Acute disseminated encephalomyelitis is often difficult to differentiate from the initial episode of MS • The cause is unknown but may represent a hypersensitivity reaction such as can occur 1–2 weeks after infection, inoculation, or chemotherapy.

Imaging Signs

▶ **Modality of choice**
MRI.

▶ **CT findings**
Multiple, subcortical, often round hypodensities that enhance with contrast.

▶ **MRI findings**
Multiple, subcortical, often round focal lesions with high signal intensity on T2-weighted images • All lesions are in the same stage, meaning that they enhance uniformly • Often there is a ring-shaped pattern of enhancement in the acute stage of inflammation • Enhancement decreases as the inflammation subsides • Occasionally bull's eye signs will be visible on T2-weighted images, lesions showing significant central hyperintensity (cystic necrosis secondary to demyelination) surrounded by moderate perifocal hyperintensity (edema).

Clinical Aspects

▶ **Typical presentation**
Similar to multiple sclerosis, although the onset of symptoms is typically abrupt and monophasic • Often accompanied by fever, meningism, mental status changes, and convulsions, which are nearly invariably absent in MS.

▶ **Treatment options**
Glucocorticoids • Plasmapheresis and cyclophosphamide may be indicated.

▶ **Course and prognosis**
Mortality of the postinfectious form is about 10–40% • Neurologic deficits often persist.

▶ **What does the clinician want to know?**
Differentiate from tumor or infarction.

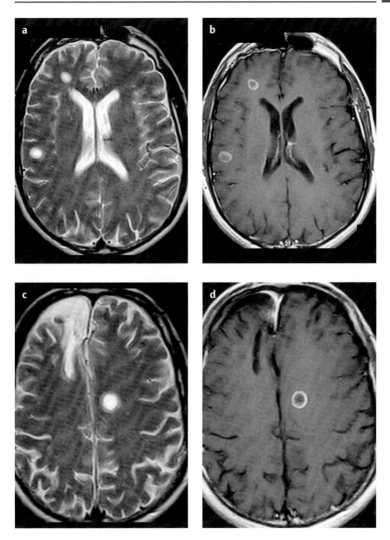

Fig. 2.5 a–d Postinfectious encephalomyelitis or acute disseminated encephalomyelitis (ADEM). Axial T2-weighted MR images (**a, c**) and axial T1-weighted MR images after contrast administration (**b, d**). Multiple subcortical hyperintensities on T2-weighted MR images that are ring-enhancing on T1-weighted MR images. Identical enhancement in all lesions (**b, d**). The patient had undergone surgery to remove an oligodendroglioma and received chemotherapy several weeks previously. Right frontal postoperative tissue defect.

Inflammation

Differential Diagnosis

Cerebral abscess	– ADC usually reduced in cystic portion
Cerebral ischemia	– Pattern of distribution corresponds to area supplied by one or more vessels
	– In acute stage is ADC invariably reduced
Parasitic disorders (such as toxoplasmosis)	– Often immunocompromised persons
	– CSF findings
Multiple sclerosis	– Predilection for periventricular white matter
Metastases and higher grade multifocal glial tumors	– Solid portion: relative regional cerebral blood volume (rrCBV) on perfusion MR images at least twice as high as in normal white matter

Tips and Pitfalls

Misinterpreting the disorder as brain tumor or metastasis.

Selected References

Hartmann M et al. Funktionelle MR-Verfahren in der Diagnostik intraaxialer Hirntumoren: Perfusions- und Diffusionsbildgebung. Rofo Fortschr Geb Rontgenstr Neuen Bildgeb Verfahr 2002; 174 (8): 955–964

Niedermayer I et al. Neuropathologische und neuroradiologische Aspekte akuter disseminierter Enzephalomyelitiden (ADEM). Radiologe 2000; 40 (11): 1030–1035

Schwarz S et al. Akute disseminierte Enzephalomyelitis (ADEM). Nervenarzt 2001; 72 (4): 241–254

Inflammation

Definition

▶ **Epidemiology**
Incidence: 1:250 000 per year. Fifty percent of the patients are younger than 50 years ● Incidence of herpes simplex encephalitis involving virus type 2 (HSV-2) in newborns is 1:200–1:5000 births.

▶ **Etiology, pathophysiology, pathogenesis**
HSV-1 encephalitis accounts for 95% of all cases; HSV-2 encephalitis occurs in 6–15% of all cases. Following primary infection the virus spreads in retrograde transneural fashion as far as the olfactory bulb or along a branch of the trigeminal nerve into the trigeminal ganglion ● There the virus persists in 70% of all patients ● Reactivation of the latent infection (for example by immunosuppression) triggers spread of the virus along the dural nerve branches into the anterior and middle cranial fossa ● Fulminant hemorrhagic, necrotizing meningoencephalitis occurs, primarily involving limbic structures (gray matter) ● Most cases of herpes simplex encephalitis in newborns are caused by HSV-2.

Imaging Signs

▶ **Modality of choice**
MRI.

▶ **CT findings**
Affected structures appear hypodense only in the advanced stages of the disorder ● Residual dystrophic calcifications will be visible.

▶ **MRI findings**
HSV-1 encephalitis: Forty-eight hours after the onset of clinical symptoms: hyperintensities on T2-weighted and FLAIR images in the medial and inferior temporal lobes extending into the insula and in the cingulate gyrus, consistent with a focal cerebral edema ● No enhancement in the early phases of the disorder ● Later, there is meningeal enhancement and a garland-shaped pattern of enhancement at the corticomedullary junction ● Parenchymal petechial hemorrhages at the corticomedullary junction, initially with high signal intensity on T1-weighted images (methemoglobin) ● Over a period of days to weeks, the contralateral hemisphere becomes involved ● After the inflammation has subsided, cystic and gliotic tissue remains with focal or diffuse brain atrophy and, rarely, dystrophic calcifications.
HSV-2 encephalitis: Unspecific swelling of the brain with cerebral edema and leptomeningeal contrast enhancement.

Inflammation

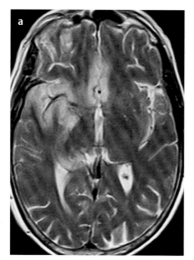 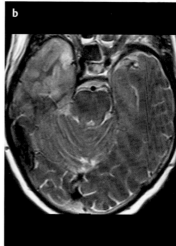

Fig. 2.6 a, b Herpes simplex virus type 1 encephalitis. Axial T2-weighted MR images. Hyperintensities in the inferior and mesial right temporal lobe, the insula, and bilaterally in the frontobasal cerebral cortex.

Clinical Aspects
....

► **Typical presentation**
HSV-1 encephalitis begins as an often asymptomatic infection of the oropharyngeal mucosa with gingivostomatitis or pharyngitis lasting 2–3 weeks ● A prodromal stage of 1–4 days follows with flu-like symptoms ● This is followed by fever, headache, disorientation, mental status changes, and convulsions.

► **Treatment options**
Specific therapy with acyclovir ● Symptomatic treatment.

► **Course and prognosis**
Mortality in untreated adults is 70%, in treated adults less than 20% ● Mortality in untreated children is 80%, in treated children 50%.

► **What does the clinician want to know?**
Differentiate from other viral encephalitides and cerebral infarctions ● Extent ● Follow-up.

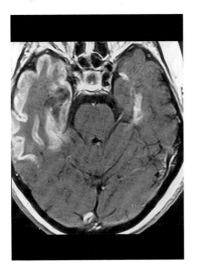

Fig. 2.7 Herpes simplex virus type 1 encephalitis. T1-weighted MR image after contrast administration. Garland-shaped hyperintensities at the corticomedullary junction from hemorrhages and contrast enhancement.

Differential Diagnosis

Low-grade multifocal or diffuse glial tumors	– No progression over a period of days – No limbic pattern of involvement
Multifocal primary cerebral lymphoma	– On perfusion MR images rrCBV is typically only moderately elevated, blood–brain barrier massively compromised, ADC reduced – No limbic pattern
ADEM	– Usually only white matter involved – No limbic pattern
Cerebral ischemia	– Pattern of distribution corresponds to the area supplied by one or more vessels – In acute stage ADC is invariably reduced – Infarcted area demarcated within days

Tips and Pitfalls

Isolated swelling of the cortex of the temporal lobe and the cingulate gyrus (an early sign as the gray matter is initially affected) is occasionally missed.

Selected References

Struffert T et al. Herpes-simplex-Virus-Enzephalitis: neuroradiologische Differenzialdiagnose. Radiologe 2000; 40 (11): 1011–1016

Definition

▶ **Epidemiology**
Incidence: approximately 1:100 000 per year • M:F = 2.3:1 • Patients with immune deficiencies or AIDS, or who have received bone marrow or organ transplants are at increased risk.

▶ **Etiology, pathophysiology, pathogenesis**
Pathogenesis: Fifty percent of all cases involve direct extension of infection (sinusitis, middle ear inflammation) • Twenty-five percent are hematogenous • Other causes: posttraumatic, foreign bodies (CSF drains).
Pathogen: Usually mixed flora • Often streptococci and staphylococci.
Localization: Junction between gray and white matter (corticomedullary junction) • Often frontal and parietal lobes.

Imaging Signs

▶ **Modality of choice**
MRI.

▶ **CT and MRI findings**
Appearance depends on the stage of the pathology (early and late cerebritis, early and late capsular stage).
  – First stage (early cerebritis, third to fifth day): On CT there is usually a subcortical hypodensity in the white matter and hyperintensity on T2-weighted images • Lesion will not necessarily enhance • Weak and expansive enhancing lesions are visualized.
  – Second stage (late cerebritis, fourth day to second week): Central hypodensity on CT and hyperintensity on T2-weighted images (necrosis) • Margin enhances • Perifocal hyperintensity on T2-weighted images (perifocal edema).
  – Third stage (early capsule formation, second week): Central hypodensity on CT and hyperintensity on T2-weighted images (necrosis) • Central necrosis often exhibits reduced ADC • Proton density- and T2-weighted images show an isointense to hypointense halo (abscess capsule) • There is a pronounced ring enhancement that is thicker closer to the surface of the brain than near the ependyma (abscess capsule) • Satellite lesions are often present.
  – Fourth stage (late capsule formation, weeks to months): Capsule collapses during further course • Edema and mass effect remit • Enhancement (scarring) can persist for a period of months • Abscesses in immunocompromised patients: capsule is thinner and enhancement less pronounced • Glucocorticoids reduce the cerebral edema and the mass effect.

Clinical Aspects

▶ **Typical presentation**
Classic triad of fever, headache, and focal neurologic deficits occurs in fewer than 50% of all patients.

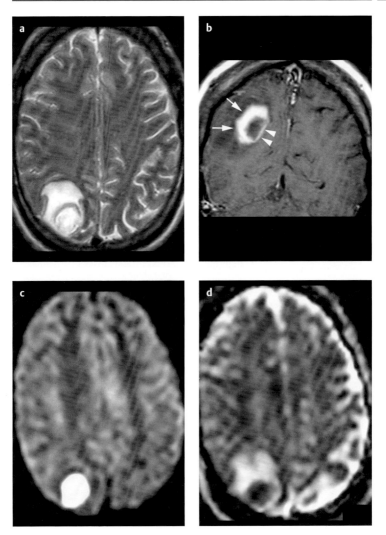

Fig. 2.8 a–d Cerebral abscess. Axial T2-weighted MR image (**a**), coronal T1-weighted MR image after contrast administration (**b**), axial diffusion-weighted MR image (**c**), and axial ADC map (**d**). Ring-enhancing structure (**b**) in the right parietooccipital region with perifocal edema (**a**). The capsule is hypointense on T2-weighted images (**a**) and is thicker close to the surface of the brain (**b**, arrows) than it is deeper within the brain, i.e., in the vicinity of the ependyma (**b**, arrowheads). Hyperintense necrosis on the diffusion-weighted image (**c**) and reduced ADC (**d**).

▶ **Treatment options**

Abscesses larger than 2.5 cm or which have a mass effect require drainage • Additional antibiotic therapy according to antibiogram • Antibiotic therapy is the sole treatment in the presence of associated meningitis, ependymitis, hydrocephalus, and risk factors contraindicating surgery • Therapy is continued for 6–8 weeks.

▶ **Course and prognosis**

Mortality even today is still 8–10% • Mortality in transplant patients is 80–90% • Most common clinical sequela is epilepsy.

▶ **What does the clinician want to know?**

Localization • Size • Satellite abscesses • Follow-up findings under therapy.

Differential Diagnosis
....

Metastases and higher grade multifocal glial tumors	– Relative regional cerebral blood volume (rrCBV) on perfusion MR images at least twice as high as in normal white matter
	– ADC in the necrotic zone usually elevated
	– MRS: high lactate concentration in tumor cysts, high amino acid concentration in untreated liquefied abscesses, high total choline concentration excludes focal inflammatory lesion; however, low total choline concentration is not diagnostic of focal inflammation
Parasitic disorders such as toxoplasmosis	– Often immunocompromised persons
	– CSF findings
Radiation necrosis	– ADC in the necrotic zone usually elevated
Hematoma in absorption	– Blood demonstrated on T2*-weighted MR images
	– History of cerebral hemorrhage
Thrombosed aneurysm	– Usually located in the circle of Willis
	– Other clinical course

Tips and Pitfalls
....

Misinterpreting as tumor or metastasis.

Selected References

Haimes AB et al. MR imaging of brain abscesses. AJR Am J Roentgenol 1989; 152 (5): 1073–1085

Hartmann M et al. Funktionelle MR-Verfahren in der Diagnostik intraaxialer Hirntumoren: Perfusions- und Diffusionsbildgebung. Röfo Fortschr Geb Röntgenstr Neuen Bildgeb Verfahr 2002; 174 (8): 955–964

Weber W et al. Septisch-embolischer und septisch-metastatischer Hirnabszess. Radiologe 2000; 40 (11): 1017–1028

Definition

▶ **Epidemiology**
Most common form of CNS infection • Incidence of lymphocytic (viral, aseptic) meningitis: 10–30:100 000 per year.

▶ **Etiology, pathophysiology, pathogenesis**
Pathogenesis: Hematogenous • Direct extension of infection (sinusitis, middle ear inflammation) • Foreign bodies (CSF drains).
Pathogen: Newborns: group B streptococci, *Escherichia coli* • Children below age 7: *Haemophilus influenzae* • Children above age 7 years: *Neisseria meningitidis* • Adults: *Streptococcus pneumoniae.*
Forms: Acute purulent (bacterial) meningitis • Lymphocytic (viral, aseptic) meningitis • Chronic (tuberculous) meningitis.

Imaging Signs

▶ **Modality of choice**
MRI.

▶ **CT findings**
Usually normal • There may be slight hydrocephalus or a hyperdense substrate in the basal cisterns (pus).

▶ **MRI findings**
Increased enhancement of the leptomeninges and occasionally the dura mater as well • Hyperintensity on T2-weighted images and on non-contrast-enhanced T1-weighted images (pus or serous effusion in the subdural or subarachnoid space) • Purulent meningitis is usually frontoparietal, tuberculous meningitis usually basal.

Clinical Aspects

▶ **Typical presentation**
Prodromal stage (hours to days) with fever, headache, and meningism • Conjunctivitis • Cranial nerve palsies.

▶ **Treatment options**
Specific antibiotic therapy • Symptomatic treatment • Glucocorticoids may be indicated to control cerebral edema • Neurosurgical decompression of subdural empyema.

▶ **Course and prognosis**
Mortality of septic meningitis 25%, morbidity 60%.
Complications: Perivascular inflammation with vasculitis and arterial or venous cerebral infarctions • Ventriculitis • Ependymitis • Occlusive or malabsorptive hydrocephalus • Subdural effusion or empyema.

▶ **What does the clinician want to know?**
Spread of the meningitis • Complications.

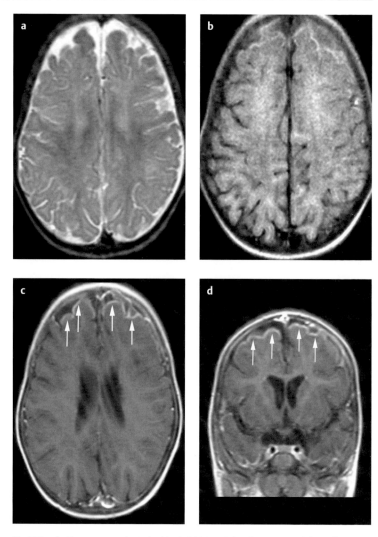

Fig. 2.9 a–d   Pneumococcal meningitis. Axial T2-weighted MR images (**a**), axial FLAIR image (**b**), and axial (**c**) and coronal (**d**) T1-weighted MR images after contrast administration. Bilateral frontopolar subdural fluid accumulations that are slightly hyperintense to CSF on T2-weighted images (**a**) and hyperintense to CSF on FLAIR images (**b**), indicative of increased protein content. Strongly enhancing thickened frontoparietal leptomeninges (**c, d**; arrows).

Differential Diagnosis

Meningeal carcinomatosis	– Contrast enhancement of the meninges often less linear and more nodular – Meninges irregularly thickened
Brain tumor (higher grade glioma, lymphoma, germinoma, pineal blastoma, ependymoma, medulloblastoma) with meningeal metastases	– Demonstrated brain tumor
CNS sarcoidosis	– Often includes cerebral parenchymal changes along the perivascular spaces
Meningeal enhancement in the setting of reduced CSF pressure	– Neuroradiologic differentiation often not possible

Tips and Pitfalls

Misinterpreting meningeal enhancement in the setting of reduced CSF pressure as meningitis.

Selected References

Coyle PK. Overview of acute and chronic meningitis. Neurol Clin 1999; 17 (4): 691–710
Pfister HW et al. Spectrum of complications during bacterial meningitis in adults. Results of a prospective clinical study. Arch Neurol 1993; 50 (6): 575–581

Definition
....

▶ **Etiology, pathophysiology, pathogenesis**

Inflammation and necrosis of the wall of cerebral blood vessels, particularly arteries • Definitive diagnosis requires biopsy, which for practical reasons is rarely performed • Exceptions: suspected temporal arteritis (transcutaneous temporal biopsy), suspected Wegener granulomatosis (biopsy of nasal mucosa) • Tentative diagnosis is based on pathologic inflammation parameters and vasculitis serology (ANCA, ANA, anti-ds-DNA) • In isolated CNS vasculitis, vasculitis serology is negative and there is no evidence of involvement of other organs.

Forms: Primary systemic vasculitis in giant cell arteritis, Wegener granulomatosis, and isolated CNS vasculitis (very rare) • Secondary vasculitides in collagen diseases such as lupus erythematosus, primary Sjögren syndrome, and scleroderma • Secondary vasculitides in infectious diseases such as bacterial meningitis, viral encephalitis, and syphilis • Secondary vasculitides in tumors or cocaine abuse.

Imaging Signs
....

▶ **Modality of choice**
DSA.

▶ **CT and MRI findings**
Depending on specific vascular involvement, ischemic infarctions occur in the areas supplied by various vessels • Inflammatory parenchymal or leptomeningeal infiltrates that enhance on T1-weighted MR images are visualized • Findings include involvement of white and gray matter, multiple arterial stenoses, occlusion or aneurysms on CT angiography or MR angiography.

▶ **DSA findings**
Best modality for demonstrating vascular changes • Multiple arterial stenoses, occlusions, or aneurysms.

Pattern of involvement: This depends on the underlying disorder:
– Aorta: Takayasu arteritis.
– Aorta and large arteries: giant cell arteritis.
– Large and medium-sized arteries: polyarthritis, Churg–Strauss angiitis.
– Medium-sized and small arteries: primary CNS vasculitis, Wegener granulomatosis, Behçet disease, Kawasaki disease.
– Small arteries and arterioles: Secondary vasculitides in collagen diseases.

Clinical Aspects
....

▶ **Typical presentation**
Cranial nerve deficits and focal neurologic symptoms, although often unspecific • Generalized symptoms such as fever, nocturnal sweating, weight loss.

▶ **Treatment options**
Treatment of the underlying disorder • Glucocorticoids and immunosuppressives (cyclophosphamide, azathioprine) • Plasmapheresis may be indicated.

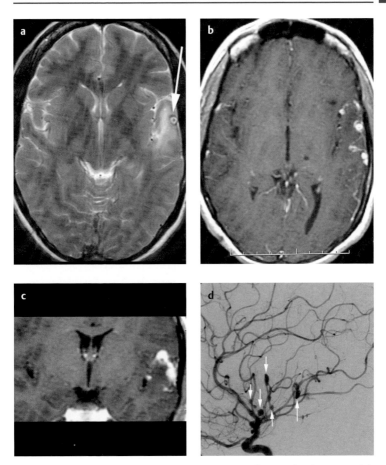

Fig. 2.10 a–d Vasculitis in circumscribed scleroderma. Axial T2-weighted MR image (**a**) and axial T1-weighted MR image after contrast administration (**b**). Coronal T1-weighted MR image after contrast administration (**c**). Lateral DSA after injection into left internal carotid artery (**d**). Broad area of hyperintensity in the left temporal operculum involving the cerebral cortex and subcortical white matter, consistent with a cerebral edema with inflammatory infiltrate (**a**, arrow). Enhancing thickened leptomeninges (**b, c**). Enhancement is also due in part to the slow blood flow in aneurysmal branches of the middle cerebral artery (**b, c**). DSA demonstrates multiple, primarily fusiform aneurysms in numerous branches of the left middle cerebral artery (**d**, arrows).

▶ **Course and prognosis**
  This depends on the cause and/or underlying disorder.
▶ **What does the clinician want to know?**
  Pattern of involvement ● Follow-up to assess the success of therapy.

Differential Diagnosis

Multiple sclerosis	– Predilection for periventricular white matter
	– Usually no involvement of gray matter
Embolic cerebral infarctions	– Differentiation only possible with vascular findings on DSA and vasculitis serology
CADASIL	– Subcortical infarctions, most often in the frontal and temporal regions (beginning in the temporopolar region) and in the inner capsule, positive family history, DNA analysis (gene defect on chromosome 19q12 from mutation of the notch 3 gene)

Tips and Pitfalls

A normal cerebral angiogram does not exclude vasculitis in small-caliber vessels as the resolution of digital subtraction angiography is only about 100–200 μm.

Selected References

Block F et al. Isolated Vasculitis of the Central Nervous System. Radiologe 2000; 40 (11): 1090–1097
Ferro JM. Vasculitis of the central nervous system. J Neurol 1998; 245 (12): 766–676

Definition

▶ **Epidemiology**
Frequency: Occurs in 15% of all AIDS patients • The most common opportunistic infection of the CNS • Second most common cause of congenital infections after cytomegalovirus infection • A high proportion of the normal population are carriers.

▶ **Etiology, pathophysiology, pathogenesis**
The pathogen is the obligatory intracellular protozoan *Toxoplasma gondii* • The most significant sources of infection are infected food and cat feces • The pathogen can also be transmitted via unpasteurized milk, body fluids, transfusions, contaminated cannulas, and organ transplants, or through the placenta to the fetus • Toxoplasmosis lesions exhibit a three-layer structure without a capsule: a necrotic center, a middle layer of inflammatory tissue, and an outer layer of pathogens in small cysts.

Imaging Signs

▶ **Modality of choice**
MRI • CT to demonstrate calcifications.

▶ **CT findings**
Enhancing hypodensities with mass effect • Calcifications.

▶ **MRI findings**
Toxoplasmosis lesions are typically hypointense or isointense on T1-weighted images and isointense to hyperintense on T2-weighted images • Localization: Subcortical white matter, usually at the corticomedullary junction, basal ganglia, and cerebral cortex • Lesions often exhibit ring enhancement due to the central necrosis • The enhancing ring is usually thin with a smooth margin • Smaller lesions may also show nodular enhancement • Lesions vary in size, 1–3 cm, often with a disproportionately large perifocal edema • Toxoplasmosis lesions in AIDS patients can also occur without edema or mass effect • Lesions may exhibit calcification and hemorrhaging under specific therapy.

Clinical Aspects

▶ **Typical presentation**
Incubation period is 3–10 days • This is followed by headache, fatigue, and focal neurologic deficits.

▶ **Treatment options**
Pyrimethamine and sulfamethoxazole.

▶ **Course and prognosis**
Progressive encephalitis that is fatal if left untreated.

▶ **What does the clinician want to know?**
Differentiate from lymphoma, fungal infection, and neurosyphilis • Follow-up.

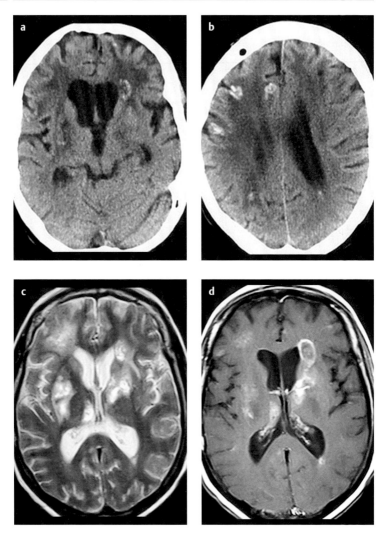

Fig. 2.11 a–d   Toxoplasmosis. Axial CT (**a, b**), axial T2-weighted MR image (**c**), and axial image after contrast administration (**d**). On CT (**a, b**) there are multiple edematous lesions, some calcified, in the basal ganglia and inner capsule on both sides (**a**), in the subcortical right hemisphere (**b**), and at periventricular locations (**b**). Toxoplasmosis lesions are more sharply delineated on T2-weighted images (**c**). The majority of the lesions show enhancing areas, some of them ring-enhancing (**d**).

Differential Diagnosis

Cerebral lymphoma	– Relative regional cerebral blood volume (rrCBV) in toxoplasmosis lesions not elevated or only elevated 50% with respect to normal values; in lymphomas rrCBV is elevated and the blood–brain barrier is massively compromised
	– ADC in toxoplasmosis lesions is significantly elevated with respect to normal values; in lymphomas it is usually lower than normal
	– No improvement with pyrimethamine and sulfamethoxazole
Other ring-enhancing lesions	– See Cerebral Abscess (p. 38)

Tips and Pitfalls

Misdiagnosing as lymphoma ● Misinterpreting finely dispersed calcifications as hemorrhage on T1-weighted MR images.

Selected References

Camacho DL et al. Differentiation of toxoplasmosis and lymphoma in AIDS patients by using apparent diffusion coefficients. AJNR Am J Neuroradiol 2003; 24 (4): 633–637

Chang KH et al. MRI of CNS parasitic diseases. J Magn Reson Imaging 1998; 8 (2): 297–307

Ernst TM et al. Cerebral toxoplasmosis and lymphoma in AIDS: perfusion MR imaging experience in 13 patients. Radiology 1998; 208 (3): 663–669

Progressive Multifocal Leukoencephalopathy (PML)

Definition

▶ **Epidemiology**
Frequency: Occurs in 4–7% of all patients with AIDS ● Most common opportunistic viral infection of the CNS ● There is also a high incidence in patients with severely compromised cellular immune response such as in leukemia, Hodgkin disease, and autoimmune disorders.

▶ **Etiology, pathophysiology, pathogenesis**
Pathogen: JC virus (papova virus containing DNA) ● JC virus attacks oligodendrocytes, leading to multifocal demyelination.

Imaging Signs

▶ **Modality of choice**
MRI.

▶ **CT findings**
Hypodensity in the affected areas.

▶ **MRI findings**
Onset: Parietooccipital subcortical white matter ● Most common localization: Parietooccipital centrum semiovale ● Arcuate fibers are invariably involved in contrast to HIV encephalopathy ● Cerebral cortex is spared.
Advanced stage: Medullary lesions have high signal intensity on T2-weighted images; these lesions become progressively larger and confluent ● Involvement of the thalamus, basal ganglia, corpus callosum, and infratentorial structures is also possible ● Lesions almost never enhance with contrast.

Clinical Aspects

▶ **Typical presentation**
Headache ● Cognitive defects ● Visual field defects ● Hemiparesis or ataxia depending on the affected structure.

▶ **Treatment options**
Symptomatic treatment ● Optimal antiviral therapy with respect to HIV.

▶ **Course and prognosis**
Usually fatal within a year of the diagnosis.

▶ **What does the clinician want to know?**
Differentiate from ADEM and HIV encephalopathy ● Follow-up.

Differential Diagnosis

HIV encephalopathy	– Arcuate fibers are not involved
ADEM	– Lesions tend to be round
	– Invariably enhancing during the acute phase
Primary cerebral lymphoma	– Blood–brain barrier is massively compromised
	– Strong enhancement
	– ADC is usually reduced

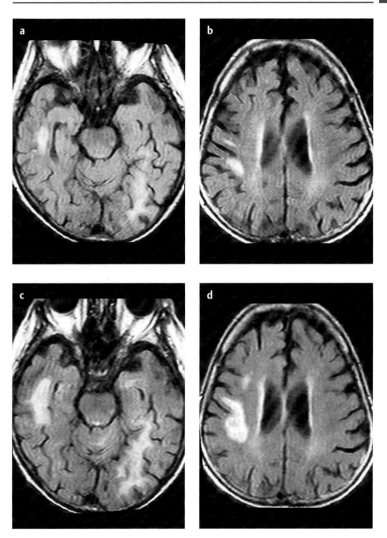

Fig. 2.12a–d Progressive multifocal leukoencephalopathy. Axial FLAIR images. Images **c** and **d** were obtained one month after images **a** and **b**. Bilateral expanding hyperintensities in the temporooccipital white matter (**a, c**) and in the right parietal region (**b, d**). In contrast to HIV encephalitis, the arcuate fibers are also involved.

Inflammation

Tips and Pitfalls
....

Misinterpreting as HIV encephalopathy.

Selected References

Post MJ et al. Progressive multifocal leukoencephalopathy in AIDS: are there any MR findings useful to patient management and predictive of patient survival? AIDS Clinical Trials Group, 243 Team. AJNR Am J Neuroradiol 1999; 20 (10): 1896–1906

Inflammation

Definition

▶ **Epidemiology**
Incidence of tuberculosis: 9:100 000 per year ● Incidence of extrapulmonary tuberculosis including CNS tuberculosis: 1–2:100 000 per year ● Occurs in 2–5% of all patients with tuberculosis and in 10% of AIDS patients with tuberculosis ● Sixty to seventy percent of patients with CNS tuberculosis are younger than 20 years of age.

▶ **Etiology, pathophysiology, pathogenesis**
CNS tuberculosis is the most severe complication of tuberculosis ● Pathogen: *Mycobacterium tuberculosis* ● CNS tuberculosis occurs primarily in AIDS patients and in patients receiving immunosuppression therapy.

Imaging Signs

▶ **Modality of choice**
MRI.
▶ **CT findings**
Only to demonstrate calcifications.
▶ **MRI findings**
Leptomeningeal tuberculosis: Enhancement of the basal meninges with hydrocephalus and cerebral infarctions in supratentorial structures and the brainstem ● Normalized enhancement of the leptomeninges is regarded as an indicator of successful therapy ● However, leptomeningeal enhancement can persist years after successful conclusion of tuberculostatic treatment ● Residual findings: meningeal or ependymal calcifications.
Dural tuberculosis: Uniformly and homogeneously enhancing lesions on the dura with mass effect ● Lesions are isointense on non-contrast-enhanced T1-weighted images and isointense to hypointense on T2-weighted images.
Parenchymal tuberculosis: Parenchymal lesions with mass effect (granulomas) that are hypointense on non-contrast-enhanced T1-weighted images and hyperintense on T2-weighted images ● Perifocal edema ● Residual findings: Calcifications or regional cerebral atrophy.
Tuberculous cerebral abscess: Radiologic appearance resembles a caseous granuloma with central necrosis, although usually larger and with a thinner wall.
Tuberculous encephalopathy: Extensive cerebral edema, occasionally involving both hemispheres.
▶ **DSA findings**
In tuberculous leptomeningitis, these include vascular stenoses due to vasculitis.

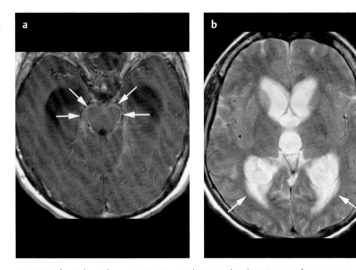

Fig. 2.13 a, b Tuberculous meningitis. Axial T1-weighted MR image after contrast administration (**a**) and axial T2-weighted MR image (**b**). Increased enhancement and thickening of the basal leptomeninges (**a**, arrows) with hydrocephalus (**b**) and CSF expressed through the ependyma. This is most obvious around the posterior horns of the lateral ventricles (**b**, arrows).

Clinical Aspects

▶ **Typical presentation**
   Tuberculous leptomeningitis: Fever ● Headache ● Mental status changes ● Signs of meningeal irritation ● Basal cranial nerve deficits.
   Parenchymal tuberculosis: Clinical findings are less pronounced than in meningeal tuberculosis ● Fever may or may not be present.
   Tuberculous cerebral abscess: Rapid clinical course with fever, headache, and focal neurologic deficits.

▶ **Treatment options**
   Standard therapy: Isoniazid, rifampicin, and ethambutol ● In endemic areas, treatment may be expanded to include pyrazinamide and streptomycin.

▶ **Course and prognosis**
   The course depends on pathogen resistance and the underlying disorder ● Severe clinical courses with hydrocephalus and paraplegia have become rare since the introduction of tuberculostatic therapy ● Tuberculous encephalopathy: usually fatal within 1–2 months despite tuberculostatic therapy.

▶ **What does the clinician want to know?**
   Differentiate basal tuberculous meningitis from bacterial meningitis ● Follow-up under therapy.

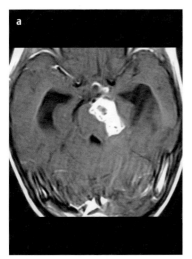 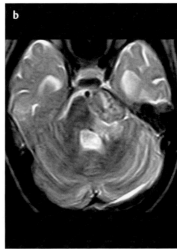

Fig. 2.14 a, b Tuberculous granuloma. Axial T2-weighted MR image (**a**) and axial T1-weighted MR image after contrast administration (**b**). Inhomogeneous hypointense signal on T2-weighted images characteristic of tuberculous granulomas.

Differential Diagnosis

Nontuberculous bacterial (pyogenic) cerebral abscess	– MRS: increased concentrations of amino acids, acetates, and succinates in pyogenic cerebral abscesses – MRS: only increased concentrations of lipids and lactates in tuberculous abscesses
Other infectious diseases such as nontuberculous bacterial meningitides or fungal diseases	– Culturing and identifying the pathogen, Mycobacterium tuberculosis
Metastases and higher grade multifocal glial tumors	– Relative regional cerebral blood volume (rrCBV) on perfusion MR images at least twice as high as in normal white matter – ADC in the necrotic zone usually elevated – MRS: high lactate concentration in tumor cysts, high amino acid concentration in untreated liquefied abscesses – MRS: high total choline concentration excludes focal inflammatory lesion; however, low total choline concentration is not diagnostic of focal inflammation

Inflammation

Tips and Pitfalls

Misinterpreting a new enhancing lesion under effective tuberculostatic therapy as progression of the disease ● Cause of this phenomenon: tubercle bacilli destroyed by medication increasingly release tuberculoprotein, triggering an inflammatory reaction.

Selected References

Bernaerts A et al. Tuberculosis of the central nervous system: overview of neuroradiological findings. Eur Radiol 2003; 13 (8): 1876–1890

Shah GV. Central nervous system tuberculosis: imaging manifestations. Neuroimaging Clin N Am 2000; 10 (2): 355–374

Definition

▶ **Epidemiology**
The world's most common parasitic infection of the central nervous system ● Endemic in Central and South America, eastern Europe, Africa, and Asia ● Also affects persons with normal immune systems ● CNS involvement is present in 60–90% of all cysticercosis patients.

▶ **Etiology, pathophysiology, pathogenesis**
Pathogen: Pork tapeworm (*Taenia solium*) ● Humans are normally the final host (by ingesting cysticerci in meat), pigs the intermediate host (by ingesting eggs) ● In cysticercosis, humans are the intermediate host (by ingesting eggs) ● The parasite may be transmitted in contaminated water or food (vegetables fertilized with raw feces) in poor hygienic conditions ● Localization: within the parenchyma (at the gray matter–white matter junction), ventricles, and subarachnoid space.

Imaging Signs

▶ **Modality of choice**
MRI.

▶ **MRI findings**
The radiologic picture of parenchymal cysticercosis of the brain depends on the stage.
Initial stage (simple vesicle): Focal cerebral edema is present during tissue invasion ● There may be brief enhancement, followed by development of a simple cyst (hypodense on CT, hypointense on T1-weighted images and hyperintense on T2-weighted images) ● A nodule along the wall (isodense on CT, isointense on MRI) within the cyst represents the scolex ● Minimal or absent edema.
Colloid vesicle stage: Edema ● Ring enhancement (fibrous capsule).
Granular and nodular stage: Calcified scolex ● Receding edema ● Ring enhancement.
Calcified and nodular stage: Small calcified nodules ● No enhancement ● No edema.
Cisternal and intraventricular cysticercosis of the brain: Multilobular cystic mass isointense to CSF in the basal cisterns, sylvian fissure, or ventricles, which may be mobile ● No scolex ● No enhancement around the cysts.

Clinical Aspects

▶ **Typical presentation**
This depends on the localization and stage of development ● Convulsions ● Intracranial hypertension ● Focal neurologic deficits.

▶ **Treatment options**
Anthelmintics such as praziquantel and albendazole.

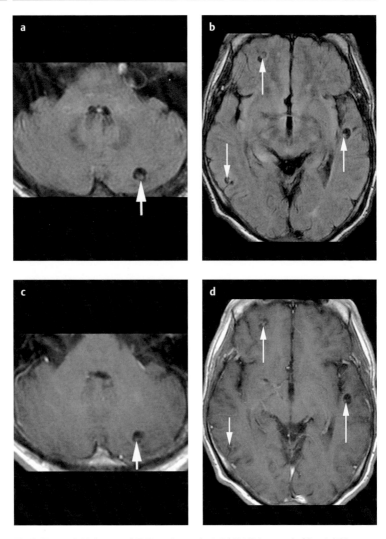

Fig. 2.15 a–e   Initial stage of CNS cysticercosis. Axial FLAIR images (**a, b**), axial T1-weighted MR images after contrast administration (**c, d**), and coronal T1-weighted MR image after IV contrast administration (**e**). Multiple lesions isointense to CSF without perifocal edema or enhancement. Tapeworm scolex within the cysts (arrows).

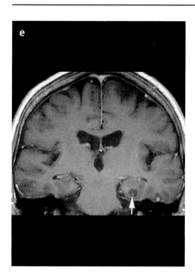

▶ **Course and prognosis**
 Prognosis under anthelmintic therapy is good • Without anthelmintic therapy
 the disorder will progress through the stages described above within 2–10 years.
▶ **What does the clinician want to know?**
 Localization • Demonstrate the scolex • Improvement of findings under therapy.

Differential Diagnosis

Metastases and higher grade multifocal glial tumors	– Relative regional cerebral blood volume (rrCBV) on perfusion-weighted MR images at least twice as high as in normal white matter – ADC in the necrotic zone usually elevated – MRS: high lactate concentration in tumor cysts, high amino acid concentration in untreated liquefied abscesses – MRS: high total choline concentration excludes focal inflammatory lesion; however, low total choline concentrations are not diagnostic of focal inflammation
Other parasitic diseases	– Scolex not demonstrated – CSF findings – Toxoplasmosis encephalitis in immunocompromised patients

Tips and Pitfalls
....

Misinterpreting findings as a brain tumor or metastasis, with neurosurgical intervention as a result.

Selected References

Chang KH et al. MRI of CNS parasitic diseases. J Magn Reson Imaging 1998; 8 (2): 297–307

Del Brutto OH et al. Proposed diagnostic criteria for neurocysticercosis. Neurology 2001; 57 (2): 177–183

Noujaim SE et al. CT and MR imaging of neurocysticercosis. AJR Am J Roentgenol 1999; 173 (6): 1485–1490

Definition

....

▶ **Epidemiology**

The most common and most severe complication of intracranial aneurysms • Incidence of aneurysmal subarachnoid hemorrhage is 4–10:100 000 per year.

▶ **Etiology, pathophysiology, pathogenesis**

Causes include ruptured aneurysm and craniocerebral trauma • Prepontine subarachnoid hemorrhage (bleeding anterior to the pons and in the perimesencephalic region with only minimal bleeding in the other CSF spaces) is due to rupture of prepontine or perimesencephalic veins.

Imaging Signs

....

▶ **Modality of choice**

CT.

▶ **CT findings**

Hyperdensity in the basal cisterns and occasionally in the peripheral CSF spaces as well, depending on the location of the ruptured aneurysm and the distribution of the blood (insular cistern, longitudinal fissure, and chiasmatic cistern) • Aneurysms of the anterior cerebral or communicating artery and posterior inferior cerebellar arteries are often accompanied by intracerebral or intracerebellar hematoma, respectively • Sensitivity of CT is 85–100% within the first 24 hours, after which it decreases.

▶ **MRI findings**

Acute subarachnoid hemorrhage: Hyperintense on T2-weighted images and isointense on T1-weighted images • Sensitivity in the acute phase for T1-weighted and T2-weighted images is only 36–50%; it is higher for proton density and FLAIR images.

Subacute subarachnoid hemorrhage (after day 5): Sensitivity of 3D FLAIR and proton density-weighted images is nearly 100% and therefore higher than CT.

Chronic subarachnoid hemorrhage: T2-weighted and proton density-weighted images show hypointensity along the adjacent leptomeninges (hemosiderin deposits, p. 244), especially on the pons and cerebellar surface and along the interpeduncular cistern.

▶ **DSA findings**

In 20% of cases initial DSA will not demonstrate an aneurysm • In prepontine subarachnoid hemorrhage, DSA will not demonstrate an aneurysm in up to 70% of cases • Vasospasm may be detected • Multiple aneurysms are present in 20% of cases (see also p. 62) • Where no aneurysm has been detected, DSA should be repeated within 10 days or when vasospasm is no longer detectable on Doppler sonography.

Fig. 3.1 Subarachnoid hemorrhage. Axial CT. Bilateral hyperdensity with blood-equivalent Hounsfield values in the basal cisterns (subarachnoid space).

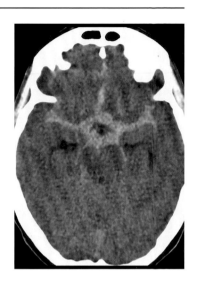

Clinical Aspects

▶ **Typical presentation**

Depends on the severity of the bleeding ● Hunt and Hess classification:
  – Grade I: Only severe headaches with abrupt onset "like never before." ● In 30% of all cases after physical exertion.
  – Grade II: Additional symptoms include stiff neck and cranial nerve palsy.
  – Grade III: Additional symptoms include slight mental status changes ● Disorientation ● Focal neurologic deficits.
  – Grade IV: Severe mental status changes ● Severe hemiparesis.
  – Grade V: Coma.

▶ **Treatment options**

Coiling or clipping the ruptured aneurysm ● Management of vasospasm ● Symptomatic treatment.

▶ **Course and prognosis**

Beginning on the third day after subarachnoid hemorrhage, vasospasm leading to cerebral ischemia may occur ● Recurrent rupture of the aneurysm with recurrent subarachnoid hemorrhage occurs in 20% of cases within 24 hours ● Communicating hydrocephalus.

▶ **What does the clinician want to know?**

Cause of the subarachnoid hemorrhage ● Is vasospasm present? ● Hydrocephalus?

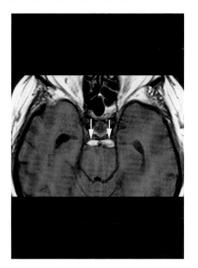

Fig. 3.2 Prepontine subarachnoid hemorrhage. Axial T1-weighted MR image. Hyperintensity in the prepontine cistern (arrows).

Differential Diagnosis

Meningitis	– Linear to patchy enhancement of the meninges – CSF findings
Meningeal carcinomatosis	– Nodular enhancement of the meninges
Contrast medium in the subarachnoid space	– Days to hours after myelography there are high density values (> 100 HU) in the entire subarachnoid space

Tips and Pitfalls

Failing to obtain four-vessel angiography to determine the cause.

Selected References

Grunwald IQ et al. Klinik, Diagnostik und Therapie der Subarachnoidalblutung. Radiologe 2002; 42 (11): 860–870

Seiler RW et al. Die Subarachnoidalblutung. Ther Umsch 1996; 53 (7): 585–589

Wiesmann M et al. Kernspintomographischer Nachweis der Subarachnoidalblutung. Röfo Fortschr Geb Röntgenstr Neuen Bildgeb Verfahr 2004; 176 (4): 500–505

Definition

▶ **Epidemiology**
Prevalence: 1–8%.
▶ **Etiology, pathophysiology, pathogenesis**
An aneurysm is dilatation of a blood vessel ● Saccular aneurysms are the most common form.
Risk factors: Family history of intracranial aneurysms ● Autosomal dominant cystic kidney disease ● Fibrous dysplasia ● Coarctation of the aorta ● Smoking.
Pathogenesis: Degeneration and weakening of the internal elastic lamina and the collagen fibers of the arterial wall ● Hemodynamic aspects.
Localization: Bifurcations or origins of the following vessels in order of frequency: anterior cerebral, middle cerebral, internal carotid, basilar, and vertebral arteries.

Imaging Signs

▶ **Modality of choice**
DSA.
▶ **CT findings**
Round to oval extra-axial hyperdensity at one of the typical locations ● An aneurysm visible on plain CT is usually larger than 5 mm ● Arterial wall calcifications ● Significant enhancement on CT after contrast administration and on CT angiography ● A partially thrombosed vessel is recognizable as a filling defect or gap in the contrast medium ● Sensitivity of CT angiography for aneurysms larger than 5 mm is about 94%; for aneurysms smaller than 5 mm it is only about 60%.
▶ **MRI findings**
The MR signal is complex because it depends on the MRI sequence and the rate and direction of blood flow ● There may be partial or complete thrombosis ● Signal loss due to blood flow (flow void) is most apparent on proton density-weighted and T2-weighted images ● The signal intensity of a suspected thrombus depends on its age ● Sensitivity of MR angiography for aneurysms larger than 5 mm is about 86%; for aneurysms smaller than 5 mm it is only about 35%.
▶ **DSA findings**
Aneurysm is visualized as a dilatation of the underlying vessel ● The precise anatomy is demonstrated (proportional relation of aneurysmal neck to sac, relationship to vessels arising from the aneurysm) ● DSA is also required to demonstrate smaller aneurysms (measuring less than 5 mm) in the presence of subarachnoid hemorrhage ● DSA aids in planning treatment and in determining whether the aneurysm can be treated by occlusion of the underlying vessel (collateral circulation).

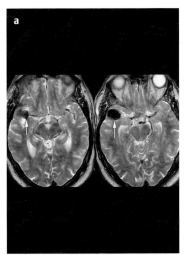

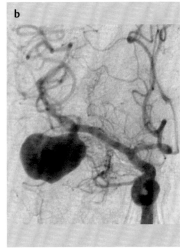

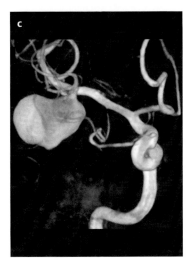

Fig. 3.3 a–c Saccular aneurysm of the trifurcation of the right middle cerebral artery. Axial T2-weighted MR image (**a**), coronal DSA after injection of the right internal carotid artery (**b**) and 3D rotational angiogram (**c**). Oval signal void originating at the main trunk of right middle cerebral artery (**a**, arrows). Vascular dilatation measuring approximately 15 mm (**b,c**).

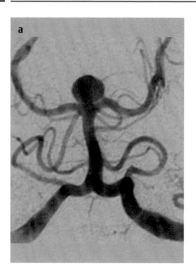 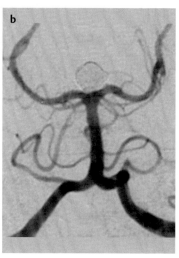

Fig. 3.4a, b Aneurysm of the tip of the basilar artery. Coronal DSA after injection of the left vertebral artery. Aneurysm measuring approximately 10 mm before (**a**) and after (**b**) endovascular embolization (coiling) with platinum coils.

Clinical Aspects

▶ **Typical presentation**
Usually asymptomatic ● Oculomotor and trochlear nerve palsy with impaired vision ● Headache ● Thromboembolic disease with ischemic stroke from partially or completely thrombosed aneurysms ● The most severe complication is rupture with subarachnoid hemorrhage.
Estimated cumulative rupture risk over 5 years:
  – Aneurysm less than 7 mm: 0% (internal carotid, anterior cerebral, middle cerebral arteries) or 2.5%, respectively (vertebral and basilar arteries).
  – Aneurysm measuring 7–12 mm: 2.6% (internal carotid, anterior cerebral, middle cerebral arteries) or 14.5%, respectively (vertebral and basilar arteries).
  – Aneurysm measuring 13–24 mm: 14.5% (internal carotid, anterior cerebral, middle cerebral arteries) or 18.4%, respectively (vertebral and basilar arteries).
  – Aneurysm larger than 24 mm: 40% (internal carotid, anterior cerebral, middle cerebral arteries) or 50%, respectively (vertebral and basilar arteries).
▶ **Treatment options**
Coiling ● Where coiling is not feasible, clipping.
▶ **Course and prognosis**
Subarachnoid hemorrhage is fatal in 30% of cases, in 30% it leads to disability, and in 30% there are no neurologic deficits.

Ruptured aneurysm: Risk of severe disability or death after coiling is about 24% ● Risk of severe disability or death after clipping is about 31%.

Unruptured aneurysm: Morbidity after coiling is about 5% ● Morbidity after clipping is about 10%.

▶ **What does the clinician want to know?**
Size ● Localization ● Number and anatomy of aneurysms.

Differential Diagnosis

Vascular sling	– Several different views with demonstration of the sling
Infundibular vascular origin	– Symmetrical origin of arising vessel
Extra-axial brain tumor (can be confused with thrombosed aneurysm)	– Thrombus usually does not enhance
Venous aneurysm in arteriovenous malformation (AVM)	– AVM demonstrated on DSA

Tips and Pitfalls

Thrombosed aneurysms on TOF MRA (without contrast enhancement) appear hyperintense like flowing blood.

Selected References

Jayaraman MV et al. Detection of intracranial aneurysms: multi-detector row CT angiography compared with DSA. Radiology 2004; 230 (2): 510–518

Molyneux A et al. International Subarachnoid Aneurysm Trial (ISAT) of neurosurgical clipping versus endovascular coiling in 2143 patients with ruptured intracranial aneurysms: a randomised trial. Lancet 2002; 360 (9342): 1267–1274

Wanke I et al. Intrakranielle Aneurysmen: Entstehung, Rupturrisiko, Behandlungsoptionen. Röfo Fortschr Geb Röntgenstr Neuen Bildgeb Verfahr 2003; 175 (8): 1064–1070

Weir B. Unruptured intracranial aneurysms: a review. J Neurosurg 2002; 96 (1): 3–42

Wiebers DO et al. Unruptured intracranial aneurysms: natural history, clinical outcome, and risks of surgical and endovascular treatment. Lancet 2003; 362 (9378): 103–110

Definition

▶ **Etiology, pathophysiology, pathogenesis**
Diffuse vascular dilatation not arising from a bifurcation or vascular origin •
Cause: Arteriosclerosis, connective-tissue disease, traumatic dissection.
Four forms are differentiated:
– Type 1: Acute dissecting aneurysms.
– Type 2: Segmental ectasia.
– Type 3: Chronic dissecting aneurysms.
– Type 4: Aneurysms at atypical locations (not at vascular bifurcations).
Histopathology: Fragmentation of the internal elastic lamina • Angiogenesis in a
thickened intima • Intramural hematoma and thrombi with vessels • Repeated
intramural hemorrhages.

Imaging Signs

▶ **Modality of choice**
DSA (CT angiography, MR angiography).
▶ **CT findings**
Tubular hyperdensity at a typical location • Fusiform aneurysm of the basilar ar-
tery: Prepontine location • Fusiform aneurysm of the middle cerebral artery:
sylvian fissure • Vascular wall calcifications • Significant enhancement after
contrast administration (CT angiography).
▶ **MRI findings**
Among other factors, the signal depends on the rate and direction of blood flow
and on the presence and age of thrombi.
▶ **DSA findings**
Shows only the patent lumen, not the thrombosed portions.

Clinical Aspects

▶ **Typical presentation/Course and prognosis**
– Types 1 and 4 (dissecting aneurysms): Risk of a rupture with subarachnoid
hemorrhage.
– Type 2: Benign course.
– Type 3: Slow enlargement, compression of adjacent structures such as the
brainstem and interventricular foramen of Monro (hydrocephalus), throm-
bosis.
▶ **Treatment options**
Thrombosis and/or stroke prophylaxis • With types 1 and 4, elimination of the
aneurysm may be indicated.
▶ **What does the clinician want to know?**
Differentiate from saccular aneurysm • Change in size • Thrombosis.

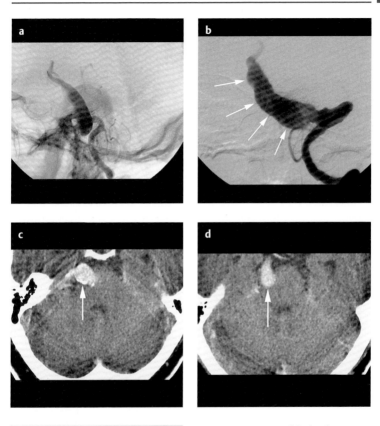

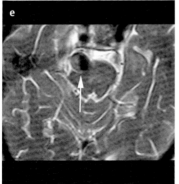

Fig. 3.5 a–e Ectasia of the basilar artery. Lateral DSA after injection of the left vertebral artery, before subtraction (**a**) and after subtraction (**b**). Axial CT after contrast administration (**c, d**) and axial T2-weighted MR image (**e**). Fusiform dilatation and stretching of the basilar artery with calcifications of the arterial wall (**b, c**, arrows) and impression of the brainstem (**d, e**).

Differential Diagnosis

Saccular aneurysm	– Differentiation with DSA
	– 3D rotational angiography may also be indicated

Tips and Pitfalls

Thrombosed aneurysms on TOF MRA (without contrast enhancement) appear hyperintense like flowing blood.

Selected References

Anson JA. Treatment strategies for intracranial fusiform aneurysms. Neurosurg Clin N Am 1998; 9 (4): 743

Mizutani T et al. Proposed classification of nonatherosclerotic cerebral fusiform and dissecting aneurysms. Neurosurgery 1999; 45 (2): 253–9; discussion 259–260

Nakatomi H et al. Clinicopathological study of intracranial fusiform and dolichoectatic aneurysms: insight on the mechanism of growth. Stroke 2000; 31 (4): 896–900

Definition

▶ **Epidemiology**
Frequency: 0.5% of the population ● Multiple cavernous hemangiomas in 15% of these cases.

▶ **Etiology, pathophysiology, pathogenesis**
Sinusoidal spaces lined with a single-cell layer of epithelium ● A collagenous stroma separates the spaces ● No brain parenchyma between the spaces ● Gliosis in the surrounding brain parenchyma ● Hemosiderin inclusions are present due to microhemorrhages ● Localization: of these lesions, 63–81% occur at supratentorial locations in the white matter; infratentorial lesions most commonly occur in the pons ● In approximately 25% of all cases, there is associated venous dysplasia or other vascular malformation such as capillary telangiectasia (immediately adjacent to the cavernous hemangioma or at another site) ● Knowledge of additional vascular malformations is important in planning neurosurgical intervention.

Imaging Signs

▶ **Modality of choice**
MRI.

▶ **CT findings**
Only large cavernous hemangiomas are demonstrated or lesions with acute hemorrhages or calcifications ● Contrast administration (double or triple dose) increases sensitivity.

▶ **MRI findings**
Central lesion may have homogeneous signal on T1- and T2-weighted images ● "Mulberry," honeycomb, or popcorn-like structure ● Lesions may enhance ● Blood in various stages of breakdown ● Perifocal edema usually occurs only with acute hemorrhage ● T2-weighted images usually show a hypointense halo, consistent with hemosiderin ● T2*-weighted images can demonstrate additional smaller cavernous hemangiomas.

▶ **DSA findings**
Cavernous hemangiomas usually occult.

Clinical Aspects

▶ **Typical presentation**
Patient usually has seizures ● There may be other focal neurologic deficits depending on the location of the lesion.

▶ **Treatment options**
Preventative surgery is not indicated ● Neurosurgical removal of the hemangioma is indicated to treat neurologic deficits due to hemorrhage and where conservative therapy fails to control seizures.

▶ **Course and prognosis**
The risk of an often asymptomatic hemorrhage is approximately 3% per patient per year and approximately 1.4–2.5% per lesion per year ● Risk factors for hemorrhage include female sex and infratentorial location.

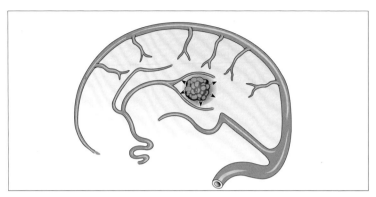

Fig. 4.1 Schematic diagram of a cavernous hemangioma. Lobular arrangement of sinusoidal spaces with hemorrhages in various stages of breakdown. The lesion is surrounded by a hemosiderin halo (arrows).

▶ **What does the clinician want to know?**

Localization ● Acute hemorrhage? ● Multiple cavernous hemangiomas? ● Association with venous dysplasia or high flow arteriovenous malformation.

Differential Diagnosis

Capillary telangiectasia	– Expansive, brushlike, or stippled structure
	– No hemosiderin halo
	– No gliosis in interposed brain tissue
Abscess	– Ring enhancement
	– Perifocal edema
	– No continuous hemosiderin rim
	– Abscess capsule hypointense on T2-weighted MR images
Metastasis	– Solid or ring enhancement, perifocal edema, no continuous hemosiderin rim
Venous dysplasia	– Converging, umbrella-like or stellar structures coursing through the cerebrum, appearing hypointense on proton density and T2-weighted MR images, hyperintense on T1-weighted images after contrast administration
Enhancing plaque in multiple sclerosis	– Typical localizationn periventricular region
	– Always hyperintense on T2-weighted images
Congophilic angiopathy	– Microangiopathy
	– No "mulberry" appearance

Tips and Pitfalls

Misinterpreting as congophilic angiopathy, which is also associated with microhemorrhages.

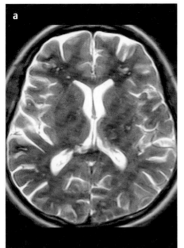

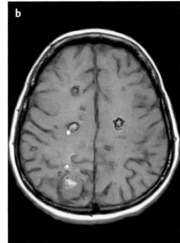

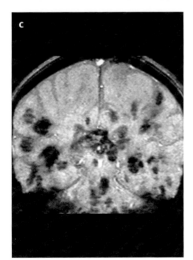

Fig. 4.2a–c Cavernous hemangioma. Axial T2-weighted MRI image (**a**), axial T1-weighted MR image (**b**), and coronal T2*-weighted MR image (**c**). Multiple homogeneous lesions with blood in all stages of breakdown (**a, b**), most showing a continuous hypointense rim on T2-weighted images (**a**) and a signal void on T2*-weighted images (**c**).

Selected References

Bertalanffy H et al. Cerebral cavernomas in the adult. Review of the literature and analysis of 72 surgically treated patients. Neurosurg Rev 2002; 25 (1–2): 1–53; discussion 54–55

Forsting M et al. Radiologie der zerebralen Gefäßmißbildungen. Aktuelle Radiol 1994; 4 (5): 209–217

Definition

▶ **Epidemiology**
Congenital vascular malformation • High incidence of 2.5% of the population (radiologic findings).

▶ **Etiology, pathophysiology, pathogenesis**
Etiology: Presumably disorganization and/or interrupted maturation of the cerebral venous system • Associated with additional vascular malformations in 19% of all cases • Associated with cavernous hemangiomas in 11% of all cases (evidence of a common genetic predisposition) • Rarely associated with arteriovenous shunt.
Localization: Frontal lobes (56% of all cases) • Cerebellum (27%).
Pathology: Veins of varying caliber • Wall thickening due to muscular hyperplasia and hyalin inclusions • Vascular architecture: proliferation of venules creating a pattern resembling the head of the Medusa; the venules drain into one or more collecting veins that course through the cerebrum • Normal brain tissue is interposed.

Imaging Signs

▶ **Modality of choice**
MRI.

▶ **CT findings**
Usually normal • Occasionally the collecting vein coursing through the cerebrum is demonstrated as a tubular hyperdensity even on non-contrast-enhanced CT images • Veins coursing in an umbrella-shaped or stellar pattern are delineated after contrast administration.

▶ **MRI findings**
Converging, umbrella-like or stellar structures coursing through the cerebrum, appearing hypointense on proton density and T2-weighted images, hyperintense on T1-weighted images after contrast administration.

▶ **DSA findings**
The arterial and parenchymal phases of the angiogram are normal • Circulation time is normal • The venous phase shows abnormally expanded intracerebral veins that collect the blood from an area of small medullary nerves.

Clinical Aspects

▶ **Typical presentation**
Asymptomatic • Where neurologic deficits are present, their symptoms should not be attributed to the venous malformation.

▶ **Treatment options**
Harmless incidental finding without clinical or therapeutic relevance unless associated with other vascular malformations.

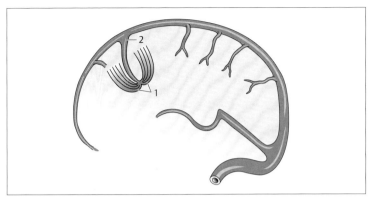

Fig. 4.3 Schematic diagram of venous dysplasia. Umbrella-like pattern of medullary veins (1) that drain into an expanded transcortical collecting vein (2).

▶ **Course and prognosis**
Risk of intracerebral hemorrhage is very slight (0.15% per lesion per year) even in the presence of an arteriovenous shunt.
▶ **What does the clinician want to know?**
Localization ● Associated cavernous hemangioma.

Differential Diagnosis

Capillary telangiectasia	– Expansive, brushlike, or stippled structure
	– Usually enhances weakly
Cavernous hemangioma	– Hemosiderin halo
	– Usually round
	– Signal inhomogeneity on T2- and T1-weighted MR images

Tips and Pitfalls

Missing a cavernous hemangioma at another location in the brain parenchyma.

Selected References

Forsting M et al. Radiologie der zerebralen Gefäßmißbildungen. Aktuelle Radiol 1994; 4 (5): 209–217

Komiyama M et al. Venous angiomas with arteriovenous shunts: report of three cases and review of the literature. Neurosurgery 1999; 44 (6): 1328–1334; discussion 1334–1335

Naff NJ et al. A longitudinal study of patients with venous malformations: documentation of a negligible hemorrhage risk and benign natural history. Neurology 1998; 50 (6): 1709–1714

Fig. 4.4 Venous dysplasia. Axial T1-weighted MR image after contrast administration. Umbrella-like pattern of veins that course through the right frontal cerebrum and drain into a larger caliber collecting vein (arrow).

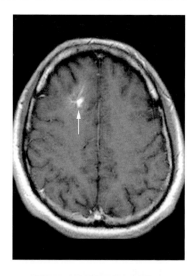

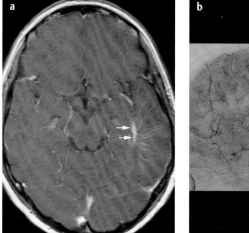

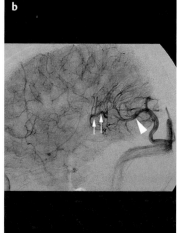

Fig. 4.5 a, b Axial T1-weighted MR image after contrast administration (**a**) and lateral DSA after injection of the left internal carotid artery (venous phase, **b**). Several small caliber veins that drain into a larger-caliber collecting vein (**a, b**; arrows). Drainage into the temporooccipital vein of Labbé (**b**, arrowhead).

Definition

▶ **Epidemiology**
Congenital vascular malformation ● High incidence of 16–20% of the population (histologic findings).

▶ **Etiology, pathophysiology, pathogenesis**
Etiology: Uncertain ● Presumably acquired, not congenital ● Possibly a sequela of impaired venous drainage.
Pathology: Numerous thin-walled elastic capillaries interspersed with normal brain tissue ● Calcification ● Gliosis ● Usually no hemorrhages ● Size: a few millimeters to 2 cm ● Localization: most frequently in the pons, less often in cerebral and cerebellar hemispheres and spinal cord ● Occasionally occurs in association with other vascular malformations such as venous dysplasia, pial arteriovenous malformations (AVM), or cavernous hemangiomas; in such a case it may be referred to as a "transitional malformation."

Imaging Signs

▶ **Modality of choice**
MRI.
▶ **CT findings**
Almost invariably normal.
▶ **MRI findings**
Hypointense to isointense on T1-weighted images ● Isointense to hyperintense on T2-weighted images ● Hypointense on T2*-weighted images (probably deoxyhemoglobin in slowly flowing blood) ● Contrast-enhanced images usually show a weakly enhancing area with a brushlike or stippled appearance ● Often associated with a large draining vein ("transitional malformation").
▶ **DSA findings**
Invariably normal except where associated malformations are present.

Clinical Aspects

▶ **Typical presentation**
Almost invariably asymptomatic.
▶ **Treatment options**
Treatment is not indicated.
▶ **Course and prognosis**
Cerebral hemorrhage occurs only in the presence of associated malformation.
▶ **What does the clinician want to know?**
Confirm findings by differential diagnosis ● Exclude inflammatory or neoplastic lesions that also enhance.

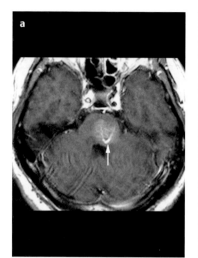

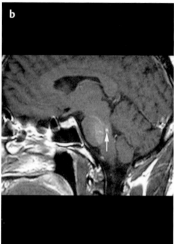

Fig. 4.6 a–c   Capillary telangiectasia. Axial T1-weighted MR image after contrast administration (**a**), sagittal T1-weighted MR image after contrast administration (**b**), and axial T2*-weighted MR image (**c**). The contrasted image shows both area enhancement and a brushlike structure in the pons (**a, b**). Hypointensity on T2-weighted images (**c**). Tubular, strongly enhancing structure in the immediate vicinity (draining vein; **a, b**; arrows).

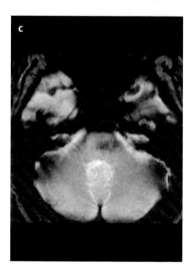

Differential Diagnosis

Cavernous hemangioma	– Hemosiderin halo – Usually round – Signal inhomogeneity on T2- and T1-weighted MR images
Abscess	– Ring enhancement – Perifocal edema – No continuous hemosiderin rim – Abscess capsule hypointense on T2-weighted MR images
Metastasis	– Solid or ring enhancement – Perifocal edema – No continuous hemosiderin rim
Venous dysplasia	– Converging, umbrella-like or stellar structures coursing through the cerebrum, appearing hypointense on proton density- and T2-weighted MR images – Hyperintense on T1-weighted MR images after contrast administration
Enhancing plaque in multiple sclerosis	– Typical localization: periventricular region – Always hyperintense on T2-weighted images

Tips and Pitfalls

Misinterpreting enhancement as enhancing inflammatory or neoplastic lesion.

Selected References

Forsting M et al. Radiologie der zerebralen Gefäßmißbildungen. Aktuelle Radiol 1994; 4 (5): 209–217

Castillo M et al. MR imaging and histologic features of capillary telangiectasia of the basal ganglia. AJNR Am J Neuroradiol 2001; 22 (8): 1553–1555

Kuker W et al. Presumed capillary telangiectasia of the pons: MRI and follow-up. Eur Radiol 2000; 10 (6): 945–950

Vascular Malformations

Definition

▶ **Epidemiology**
Prevalence: approximately 0.1% of the population ● *Peak age:* 20–40 years ● Second most common cause of stroke in young patients after cerebral aneurysms ● Rare in newborns; practically never found in fetuses ● Therefore presumably not congenital but acquired during the course of development.

▶ **Etiology, pathophysiology, pathogenesis**
Local arteriovenous shunt in the pia mater without a normal capillary bed between the two vessels ● This results in increased pressure on the nidus and draining veins (high flow AVM) ● Localization: 85% of lesions are supratentorial, 15% infratentorial ● The AVM may be fistulous or plexiform depending on the nature of the shunt ● Special form: malformation of the great vein of Galen (fistulous AVM with multiple arteries communicating with the great vein of Galen, which is often enormously expanded).
Grading with Spetzler–Martin point system:
– Size < 3 cm, 1 point; 3–6 cm, 2 points; > 6 cm, 3 points
– The surrounding brain tissue is unremarkable, 0 points; surrounding brain tissue is abnormal, 1 point
– Only superficial venous drainage, 0 points; deep venous drainage, 1 point

Imaging Signs

▶ **Modality of choice**
DSA.

▶ **CT findings**
Findings usually include a hyperdense tangle of vessels ● The inner or outer cerebral veins are enlarged ● Calcification may be present ● There is no mass effect except secondary to acute hemorrhage ● Contrast-enhanced images show a garland-like pattern of enhancement.

▶ **MRI findings**
Flow voids appearing as garland-like hypointensities are best visualized on T2-weighted and proton density-weighted images ● Adjacent brain tissue is hyperintense on T2-weighted images due to chronic ischemia (steal phenomenon) ● The draining veins in particular enhance significantly.

▶ **DSA findings**
DSA is indicated to confirm the diagnosis, visualize vascular architecture, and aid in planning treatment ● Arterial feeders are enlarged ● Veins drain prematurely and are usually enlarged ● A tangle of vessels lies between the feeders and the draining veins ● Arterial or venous aneurysms or stenoses of the draining veins may be present ● Highly selective probing of individual feeders may be indicated ● In acute hemorrhage with mass effect, hematoma can mask an AVM.

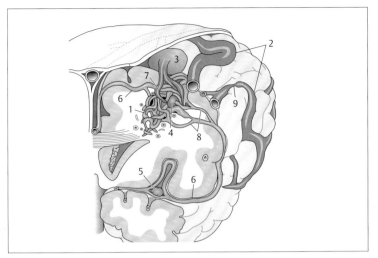

Fig. 4.7 Schematic diagram of a pial arteriovenous malformation.
1 Nidus
2 Expanded cortical vein
3 Aneurysm of the draining vein
4 Aneurysm within the nidus
5 Arterial aneurysm
6 Artery (feeder)
7 Arteriovenous fistula
8 Arterial stenosis
9 Venous stenosis

Clinical Aspects

▶ **Typical presentation**
  Intracerebral hemorrhage with a risk of 3–4% per year ● Risk of hemorrhage increases after age 55 ● Seizures occur in 45–70% of all cases ● Headache ● Hemodynamic steal phenomenon with focal hypoxemia.

▶ **Treatment options**
  Endovascular embolization with fibrin glue ● Neurosurgical removal of the AVM (according to Spetzler–Martin grading) ● Radiation therapy ● Combined therapy ● The value of treatment is questionable with grade IV and V lesions according to the Spetzler–Martin classification.

▶ **Course and prognosis**
  Mortality after initial hemorrhage is 10–18% ● Risk of recurrent bleeding after initial hemorrhage is 6–7% in the first year.

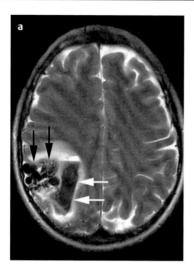

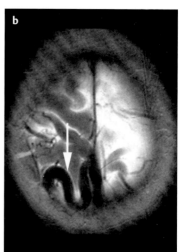

Fig. 4.8 a–c Pial arteriovenous malformation. Axial T2-weighted MR images (**a**, **b**). Lateral DSA after injection of the right internal carotid artery (**c**). Tubular flow voids in the nidus of the AVM (black arrows) on the T2-weighted images (**a**). Hypointense hematoma on T2-weighted images (deoxyhemoglobin; **a**, white arrows). Tubular signal void on the surface of the brain (vein; **b**, arrow). An early enhancing superficial cerebral vein arising from the branches of the middle cerebral artery (**c**, arrow) is seen with an interposed tangle of vessels (nidus, **c**).

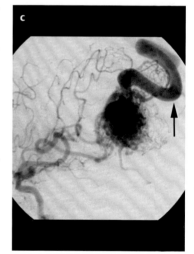

▶ **What does the clinician want to know?**
Classification of the AVM ● Vascular anatomy ● Differentiation between fistulous and nidal AVM.

Differential Diagnosis
....

Arteriovenous dural fistula	– Shunt in the dura mater
Malignant glioma with arteriovenous shunt	– Solidly enhancing – Typical growth pattern

Tips and Pitfalls
....

Missing an AVM during the phase of acute hemorrhage with mass effect.

Selected References

Fleetwood IG et al. Arteriovenous malformations. Lancet 2002; 359 (9309): 863–873
Han PP et al. Intention-to-treat analysis of Spetzler-Martin grades IV and V arteriovenous malformations: natural history and treatment paradigm. J Neurosurg 2003; 98 (1): 3–7
Soderman M et al. Management of patients with brain arteriovenous malformations. Eur J Radiol 2003; 46 (3): 195–205

Definition

▶ **Epidemiology**
Incidence: 10–15% of all intracranial arteriovenous vascular malformations •
Most common localizations: transverse sinus (50%) and cavernous sinus (16%).

▶ **Etiology, pathophysiology, pathogenesis**
Local arteriovenous shunt in the dura (sinus wall, venous plexus of the skull
base, site where cortical veins drain into a venous sinus).
Etiology is unknown; occurrence is presumably secondary to an acquired disor-
der of the affected dural sinus such as inflammation, thrombosis, or trauma.
Classification and treatment planning (Djindjian and Merland):
  – Type I: Drainage into the venous sinus with normal flow direction (no reflux)
  – Type II: Drainage into the venous sinus with reflux into other sinus or veins
  – Type IIa: Reflux into adjacent sinus
  – Type IIb: Reflux into cortical veins
  – Type III: Direct drainage into cortical veins
  – Type IV: As in type III, but with dilated varicose veins
  – Type V: Cranial fistulas with perimedullar venous or radiculomedullary drain-
    age

Imaging Signs

▶ **Modality of choice**
DSA.
▶ **CT and MRI findings**
Usually negative • Often there is partial or complete thrombotic occlusion of the
affected venous sinus • Rarely the artery feeding the fistula is expanded or there
is arterial blood flow in the draining veins.
▶ **DSA findings**
One arterial feeder, several feeders, or fistula arising directly from a large artery
such as the internal carotid artery. These often supply the dural sinus via a diffuse vascular network, causing it to enhance prematurely • Depending on the
type of fistula, the cortical veins or the superior ophthalmic vein will also enhance.

Clinical Aspects

▶ **Typical presentation**
Depending on the type of fistula, it may be asymptomatic or produce functional
symptoms such as ringing in the ears (type I); elevated intracranial pressure (diminished visual acuity, chemosis, protrusion of the globe, headache, tonsillar
herniation; type IIa); or focal neurologic deficits, myelopathy, and intracerebral
bleeding (types IIb, IIa and b, and III–V).

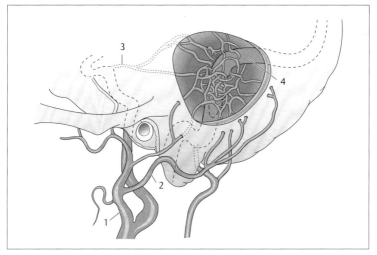

Fig. 4.9 Schematic diagram of an occipital cranial dural arteriovenous fistula. The fistula is fed by several branches of the external carotid artery (1), including the expanded occipital artery (2), and by the meningohypophyseal trunk (3) from the internal carotid artery. Drainage of the fistula into the sigmoid sinus (4).

▶ **Treatment options**
   – Type I: No treatment or nonaggressive therapy (manual vascular compression, arterial embolization)
   – Type II a: Arterial embolization or endovascular sinus occlusion
   – Types II b, II a and b, III – V: Where possible, complete obliteration of the fistula by endovascular sinus occlusion or arterial embolization; neurosurgical resection of the fistula where indicated
▶ **Course and prognosis**
   Lesions recur in up to 70% of patients treated with partial arterial embolization ● The prognosis is good for complete obliteration of the fistula.
▶ **What does the clinician want to know?**
   Confirm and localize the fistula ● Visualize all feeders ● Identify type of fistula.

Fig. 4.10 Occipital dural arteriovenous fistula. Lateral DSA after injection of the left common carotid artery. Premature filling of the transverse sinus (arrowhead) from a vascular network fed by the expanded occipital artery (arrow).

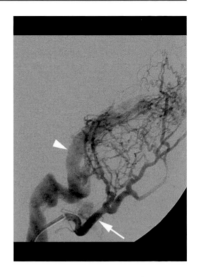

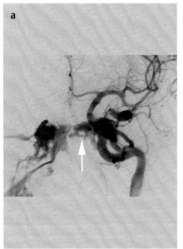

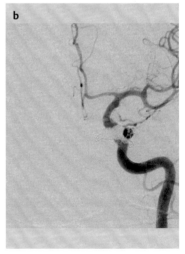

Fig. 4.11 a, b Traumatic fistula between the carotid artery and cavernous sinus before (**a**) and after (**b**) endovascular therapy. Coronal DSA after injection of the left internal carotid artery. Fed by the internal carotid artery, the left cavernous sinus enhances prematurely, as does the right cavernous sinus (**a**) as contrast-medium enters via the intercavernous sinus (arrow). Normal angiogram (**b**) after embolization of the fistula with platinum coils.

Differential Diagnosis
....

Pial AVM	– Arteriovenous "short circuit" in the pia mater
Glomus tumors	– Typical MRI findings with tumor-like "solid" enhancement and typical "salt and pepper" pattern
	– Localization: extracranial carotid bifurcation (carotid body), superior ganglion (jugular ganglion) or inferior ganglion (nodose ganglion) of the vagus nerve, tympanum

Tips and Pitfalls
....

Failing to visualize all feeders.

Selected References

Cognard C et al. Cerebral dural arteriovenous fistulas: clinical and angiographic correlation with a revised classification of venous drainage. Radiology 1995; 194 (3): 671–680

Dietrich U et al. Durafisteln mit intrakranieller Blutung: Diagnostische und therapeutische Aspekte. Zentralbl Neurochir 2003; 64 (1): 12–18

Hähnel S et al. MR appearance of an intracranial dural arteriovenous fistula leading to cervical myelopathy. Neurology 1998; 51 (4): 1131–1135

Mayer TE et al. Diagnostik und Therapie kranialer arteriovenöser Durafisteln. Radiologe 1999; 39 (10): 876–881

Definition

▶ **Etiology, pathophysiology, pathogenesis**
In itself, this is a harmless incidental finding • Usually it occurs as a result of fusion of two arteries during embryonic development or persistence of important embryonic arteries • However, such findings are often associated with cerebral aneurysms, including those located elsewhere in the cerebrovascular system.

Imaging Signs

Most variants of vascular anatomy can be demonstrated on MR angiography and CT angiography • Smaller arterial fenestrations are only detectable by DSA.

– Agenesis of the internal carotid artery. Incidence: 0.01% of the population.
– Aberrant course of the tympanic portion of the internal carotid artery.
– Unpaired (azygos) anterior cerebral artery: occurs in 0–5% of the population • The A1 segments merge into an unpaired A2 segment, which bifurcates only inferior to the free margin of the falx cerebri.
– Bihemispheric anterior cerebral artery: occurs in 2–7% of the population • The medial portions of both hemispheres are supplied by a pericallosal artery.
– Median artery of the corpus callosum: occurs in 3–22% of the population • Unpaired vessel arising from the anterior communicating artery and supplying the corpus callosum.
– Fenestration of the anterior cerebral artery: occurs in 0.1–7.2% of the population.
– Fenestration of the anterior communicating artery: occurs in 7.5–40% of the population.
– Doubled or accessory middle cerebral artery: accessory vessel arising from the internal carotid artery (doubled): occurs in 0.7–2.9% of the population. Accessory vessel arising from the anterior cerebral artery: occurs in 0.3–2.7% of the population.
– Fenestration of the basilar artery: occurs in 1–5% of the population.
– Fetal posterior cerebral artery ("embryonic origin"): occurs in 20–30% of the population • The posterior cerebral artery arises from the internal carotid artery and the P1 segment posterior cerebral artery is absent.
– Persistent primitive trigeminal artery: occurs in 0.1–1% of the population • Arises from the cavernous portion of the internal carotid artery, joining it to the basilar artery.
– Persistent primitive hypoglossal artery: occurs in 0.1–0.25% of the population • Arises from the cervical portion of the internal carotid artery and courses through the hypoglossal canal to the caudal portion of the basilar artery.
– Persistent primitive proatlantic artery: occurs in < 0.01% of the population • Type I arises from the internal or external carotid artery and courses through the foramen magnum to the distal portion of a vertebral artery (V4 segment) • Type II arises from the external carotid artery and courses to the distal portion of a vertebral artery (V3 segment).

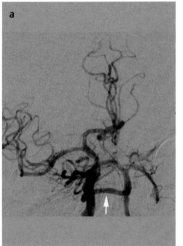 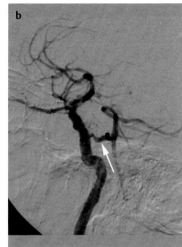

Fig. 4.12 a, b Primitive trigeminal artery (arrow). Coronal (**a**) and lateral (**b**) DSA after injection of the right internal carotid artery.

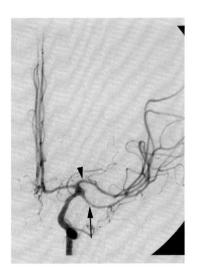

Fig. 4.13 Duplication of the middle cerebral artery. Coronal DSA after injection of the left internal carotid artery. An additional branch of the middle cerebral artery arises from the internal carotid artery, proximal to the origin of the main trunk of the left middle cerebral artery (arrowhead).

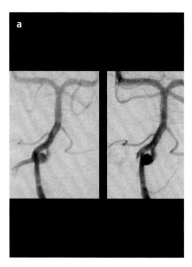 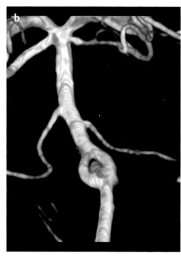

Fig. 4.14 a, b Fenestration of the basilar artery with an aneurysm at the confluence of the vertebral arteries. Coronal DSA after injection of the left vertebral artery (**a**). 3D rotation angiogram (**b**), posterior view.

Clinical Aspects

▶ **Typical presentation**
   Usually asymptomatic.
▶ **Treatment options**
   Treatment is indicated only in the presence of an associated aneurysm.
▶ **Course and prognosis**
   Usually harmless incidental findings ● Occur in association with cerebral aneurysms ● A primitive hypoglossal artery allows passage of thromboemboli from the carotid artery to the posterior circulatory system.
▶ **What does the clinician want to know?**
   Association with aneurysm.

Tips and Pitfalls

Bilateral fetal posterior cerebral artery can be mistaken for thrombosis of the basilar artery tip on intra-arterial angiography.

Selected References

Okahara M et al. Anatomic variations of the cerebral arteries and their embryology: a pictorial review. Eur Radiol 2002; 12 (10): 2548–2561

Definition

▶ **Epidemiology**
Frequency: 4.5 per million ● Women are affected more often than men ● *Peak age:* 50–70 years.

▶ **Etiology, pathophysiology, pathogenesis**
Seventy percent of all cases involve contact between an artery and a cranial nerve root at its point of entry (where there is less cushioning from Schwann cells) ● Chronic pulsation trauma leads to nerve injury.
Vessel causing symptoms:
 – Trigeminal nerve: Superior cerebellar artery or anterior inferior cerebellar artery (trigeminal neuralgia)
 – Glossopharyngeal nerve: Posterior inferior cerebellar artery or vertebral artery (glossopharyngeal neuralgia)
 – Facial nerve: Posterior inferior cerebellar artery or anterior inferior cerebellar artery (facial hemispasm)

Imaging Signs

▶ **Modality of choice**
MRI.

▶ **MRI findings**
High-resolution MRI sequences (voxel size less than 1 mm) are essential for diagnosis ● A multiplanar reconstruction is required ● The trigeminal nerve is examined in coronal slices, the facial and glossopharyngeal nerves in axial slices ● Contact between nerve and vessel (no CSF between nerve and vessel ● Nerve is displaced (twisted) ● Atrophy indicative of nerve injury is present in trigeminal neuralgia ● In 30% of cases trigeminal neuralgia is caused by inflammatory CNS disease. In these cases, there is usually no visible neurovascular impingement but there are inflammatory plaques in the brain parenchyma.

Clinical Aspects

▶ **Typical presentation**
Trigeminal neuralgia: Classic trigeminal neuralgia: brief bout of intense pain lasting a few seconds (possibly involving a trigger point) in the area supplied by the trigeminal nerve (usually V2 and V3).
Glossopharyngeal neuralgia: Brief intense unilateral pharyngeal pain associated with swallowing.
Facial hemispasm: Unilateral twitching of the musculature of the face supplied by the facial nerve.

▶ **Treatment options**
Trigeminal neuralgia: Medical therapy with an agent such as carbamazepine ● Surgical ablation: coagulation of trigeminal ganglion ● Curative surgery: Jannetta microvascular decompression.

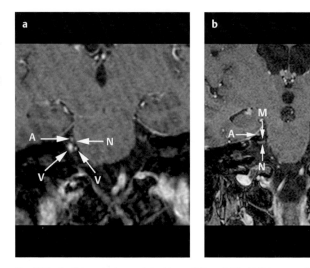

Fig. 4.15 a, b   Trigeminal neuralgia. Coronal T1-weighted MR images after contrast administration before (**a**) and after (**b**) Janetta procedure for right trigeminal neuralgia. Superior cerebral artery (A) and tentorial veins (V) are in contact with the right trigeminal nerve (N in **a**) at its point of entry. The nerve is displaced. The volume of the affected nerve is reduced compared with the normal contralateral side (**a**). The position of the Gore-Tex membrane (M) following the Jannetta procedure is well visualized (**b**, artery [A] and nerve [N] are separated).

> *Glossopharyngeal neuralgia:* Medical therapy with an agent such as carbamazepine ● Curative surgery: Jannetta microvascular decompression.
> *Facial hemispasm:* Medical therapy such as injections of botulinum toxin ● Curative surgery: Jannetta microvascular decompression.

▶ **Course and prognosis**

The Janetta procedure is curative in 80% of trigeminal neuralgia treated in this manner. No comprehensive statistics are available on glossopharyngeal neuralgia and facial hemispasm.

▶ **What does the clinician want to know?**

Neurovascular conflict ● Displacement of the nerve ● Atrophy ● Tumor ● Nerve injury ● Inflammatory CNS disorder.

Vascular Malformations

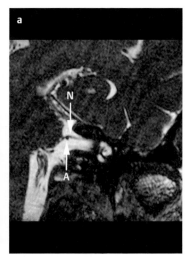
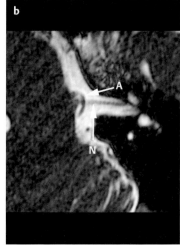

Fig. 4.16a, b Left facial nerve hemispasm. Coronal (**a**) and axial (**b**) reconstruction from a T2-weighted 3D TRUE FISP sequence. The posterior inferior cerebellar artery (A) displaces the facial nerve root (N) at its point of entry.

Differential Diagnosis

Neuropathy	– Classic history: persistent dull pain, often after extraction of a tooth
	– Include paranasal sinuses and petrous bone in the examination: perineural tumor spread can cause neuropathy
Neurinoma	– Enhancing thickening of the nerve
Meningioma	– Enhancing thickening of the meninges

Tips and Pitfalls

Not every neurovascular conflict is pathologic (are there clinical findings or nerve atrophy?) • Failing to examine the petrous bone and paranasal sinus as well • Using sequences with a voxel size larger than 1 mm.

Selected References

Jannetta PJ et al. Arterial compression of the trigeminal nerve at the pons in patients with trigeminal neuralgia J Neurosurg 1967; 26 (1) Suppl: 159–162

Majoie CB et al. Trigeminal neuralgia: comparison of two MR imaging techniques in the demonstration of neurovascular contact. Radiology. 1997; 204 (2): 455–460

Kress B et al. MR Volumetrie des N. trigeminus bei Patienten mit einseitigen Gesichtsschmerzen. Rofo Fortschr Geb Rontgenstr Neuen Bildgeb Verfahr 2004; 176 (5): 719–723

Definition

▶ **Epidemiology**
The most common cause of stroke, accounting for 70% of all cases • *Incidence:* 130:100 000 per year • Stroke is the third most common cause of death after heart attack and cancer • Incidence in children is 3–8:100 000 children per year.

▶ **Etiology, pathophysiology, pathogenesis**
 – Adults: Arteriosclerosis of the large extracranial arteries supplying the brain • Arteriosclerosis due to hypertension • Embolic vascular occlusion • Inflammatory vascular disease.
 – Newborns: Hypercoagulability in the mother.
 – Infants and young children: Vasculopathies (Moya Moya, infectious vasculitis) • Systemic disorders (inflammatory bowel disease, systemic lupus erythematosus) • Hematologic disorders (sickle-cell anemia, iron deficiency anemia, nocturnal hypoxemia) • Congenital heart defects • Metabolic disorders (MELAS, progeria, homocystinuria, neurocutaneous syndrome).
 – Older children up to age 15 years: Coagulatory disorders.
 Pathophysiologic course
 – First three days (necrotic stage): Impaired perfusion initially leads to cytotoxic cellular swelling of the perivascular astrocytes and endothelial cells (cytotoxic cerebral edema) • Destruction of the blood–brain barrier begins after six hours with a vasogenic cerebral edema • Leukocyte infiltration occurs after 24 hours.
 – Beginning on the fourth day (absorption stage): Necrotic tissue is phagocytosed • Edema becomes maximal between the third and fifth days.
 – From 10 to 30 days (organization phase): Formation of residual cysts or gliosis.

Imaging Signs

Pathogenetic classification is often possible on the basis of the typical pattern of infarction (embolic or hemodynamic infarction) • MRI is generally superior to CT for infratentorial infarctions.

▶ **Modality of choice**
Up to six hours after onset of symptoms: MRI.

Acute Brain Infarction

▶ **CT findings**
Plain CT: Early signs of infarction may be expected within two hours of the onset of symptoms: Gray matter hypodensity • Effacement of cerebral sulci • Hyperdense medial cerebral artery sign (intravascular thrombus) • Swelling of the brain.
CT angiography: Arterial occlusion.
Perfusion CT: Impaired perfusion (reduced rrCBV and rCBF and extended rMTT) in all or part of the area supplied by an artery.

▶ **MRI findings**
Acute findings: Reduced ADC (several minutes to nine days after onset of symptoms) and impaired perfusion in the area supplied by an artery • Affected arteries without flow void.

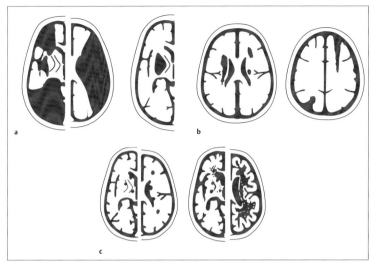

Fig. 5.1 a–c Schematic diagram of different patterns of cerebral infarction (after Ring-elstein). Territorial (embolic) infarction pattern (**a**), hemodynamic infarction pattern (watershed or border-zone infarction, **b**), and microangiopathic infarction pattern (**c**).

Up to 12 hours after onset of symptoms: Effacement of cerebral sulci • Reduced demarcation between gray and white matter on T1-weighted images.
Over 12 hours after onset of symptoms: Hyperintensity on T2-weighted images.
MR angiography: Arterial occlusion.
▶ **DSA findings**
Vessel is interrupted in the affected territory • Pial collateral vessels may be demonstrated.

Subacute and Chronic Brain Infarction

▶ **CT findings**
Hypodensity in the area supplied by an artery that initially expands (first to seventh days) and later contracts (after the seventh day) • Fogging effect (infarction appears isodense to brain tissue as a result of hyperemia and petechial hemorrhaging) occurs during the absorption stage (second to third week) • Present from the fourth day to 6–8 weeks after onset of symptoms with maximal enhancement after 1–2 weeks.
▶ **MRI findings**
Expansion and contraction of lesion and enhancement are similar to findings on CT • Hypointensity on T2-weighted images (fogging effect) may be seen in the first eight weeks • ADC increases after the ninth day.
▶ **DSA findings**
Vessels that fail to reopen are seen to be interrupted in the affected area.

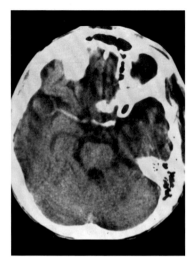

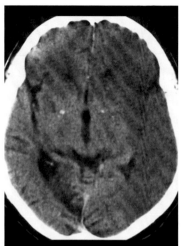

Fig. 5.2 Hyperdensity of the right middle cerebral artery as a result of thrombosis (hyperdense MCA sign).

Fig. 5.3 Subacute left middle cerebral artery infarction. Axial CT. Broad hypodensity with a slight mass effect in the entire area supplied by the left middle cerebral artery with loss of demarcation between the cortex and white matter.

Clinical Aspects

▶ **Typical presentation**
   Focal neurologic deficiency with acute onset corresponding to the location of the infarction • Brainstem infarctions and large supratentorial infarctions are also accompanied by impaired consciousness.

▶ **Treatment options**
   Acute treatment is symptomatic • Patency may be restored in the acute stage by intravenous or intra-arterial thrombolysis depending on CT or MRI findings (mismatch concept) • Secondary prophylaxis (platelet aggregation inhibitors, carotid surgery, or stenting).

▶ **Course and prognosis**
   Early mortality: 10–30% within one month • Only one-third of all patients successfully return to work and social self-sufficiency.

▶ **What does the clinician want to know?**
   Localization of the infarction • Volume of the irreversibly damaged brain tissue and penumbra of impaired profusion • Vascular occlusion • Exclude tumor, inflammation, or cerebral hemorrhage.

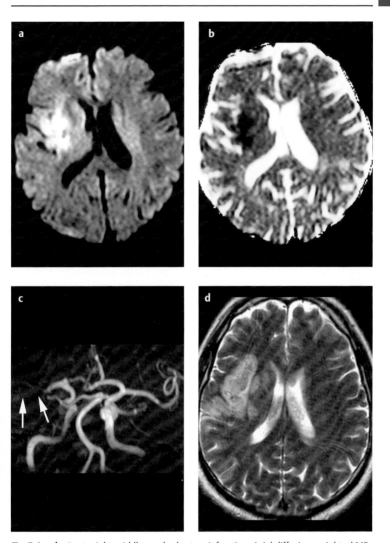

Fig. 5.4 a–d Acute right middle cerebral artery infraction. Axial diffusion-weighted MR image (**a**), axial ADC map (**b**), MIP reconstruction of an arterial MR angiogram (**c**), axial T2-weighted MR image (**d**). High signal intensity on the diffusion-weighted image (**a**) and reduced ADC (**b**; infarcted area is dark). There is no blood flow in the distal main trunk of the right middle cerebral artery (**c**; arrows). Twenty-four hours after onset of symptoms the infarction is well demarcated as a hyperintensity on T2-weighted images (**d**).

Fig. 5.5 Pons infarction. Axial T2-weighted MR image. Wedge-shaped hyperintensity in the right paramedian pons.

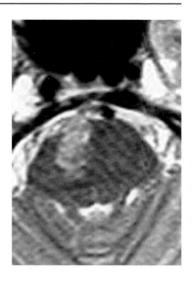

Differential Diagnosis

Encephalitis	– No territorial involvement
	– No demarcation within hours
	– ADC not reduced in the first few days
Brain tumor	– ADC usually not reduced
	– No territorial involvement
	– No demarcation within hours
Hyperdense vascular sign with elevated hematocrit	– All cranial arteries and veins are hyperdense

Tips and Pitfalls

Failing to allow for the fogging effect ● Misinterpreting increased signal intensity on diffusion-weighted MR images due to the T2 "shine-through" effect as an acute infarction: signal increase on diffusion-weighted images results from the reduced ADC and increased T2 time.

Selected References

deVeber G. Stroke and the child's brain: an overview of epidemiology, syndromes and risk factors. Curr Opin Neurol 2002; 15 (2): 133–138

Fiebach JB et al. Moderne Kernspintechniken beim Schlaganfall. Radiologe 2003; 43 (3): 251–263

Jansen O et al. Neuroradiologische Diagnostik beim akuten arteriellen Hirninfarkt: Momentaner Stellenwert neuer Verfahren. Nervenarzt 1998; 69 (6): 465–471

Definition

▶ **Epidemiology**
  Detectable in over 30% of all persons over 60 years • Associated with vascular risk factors.
▶ **Etiology, pathophysiology, pathogenesis**
  SAE: Subcortical atherosclerotic encephalopathy (SAE) or Binswanger disease • Diffuse subcortical lesions • Indicative of tissue adaptation to hypoperfusion with decreased oligodendroglia and myelin content • Localization: periventricular and subcortical white matter, sparing the arcuate fibers.
  Lacunar infarctions: Small infarctions from occlusion of the penetrating arterioles with diameters of 40–200 μm by lipid hyalin degeneration and fibrinoid necrosis • Localization: basal ganglia, thalamus, internal and external capsules, periventricular medulla, pons.

Imaging Signs

▶ **Modality of choice**
  MRI.
▶ **CT findings**
  SAE: Confluent area hypodensities in the medulla.
  Lacunae: Sharply demarcated hypodensities measuring 2–5 mm without mass effects • Located at common sites.
▶ **MRI findings**
  SAE: Confluent area hyperintensities on T1-weighted and proton density images or hypointensities in the white matter on T1-weighted images.
  Lacunae: Sharply demarcated hyperintensities measuring 2–5 mm on T2-weighted and proton density images or hypointensities without mass effects (on T1-weighted images) at the common sites mentioned above.
  Amyloid angiopathy: Multilocular microhemorrhages on T2*-weighted images.

Clinical Aspects

▶ **Typical presentation**
  Unspecific microangiopathy: Broad spectrum ranging from normal findings to acute focal neurologic deficits (acute lacuna) to vascular dementia.
  SAE: Onset is between the ages of 55 and 75 years • Focal neurologic and neuropsychologic deficits.
▶ **Treatment options**
  Elimination of risk factors such as hypertension and smoking, and treatment of diabetes mellitus.
▶ **Course and prognosis**
  SAE is characterized by episodic progression of the motor, cognitive, and behavioral deficits over a period of 5–10 years with periods of stabilization.
▶ **What does the clinician want to know?**
  Extent of the microangiopathy • Differential diagnosis.

Fig. 5.6 Subcortical atherosclerotic encephalopathy (SAE). Axial CT. Area hypodensities in the periventricular white matter.

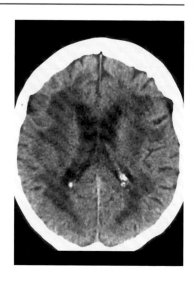

Differential Diagnosis

Multiple sclerosis	– Corpus callosum often involved – CSF findings – Younger patients
CADASIL	– Subcortical infarctions, most commonly frontal and temporal beginning in the temporopolar region) and in the inner capsule – Positive family history – DNA analysis (gene defect on chromosome 19q12 due to mutation of the notch 3 gene)
Physiologic lines of increased signal intensity in the anterior and posterior horns on FLAIR and proton density MR images	– Normal subependymal gliosis or increased interstitial water content
Virchow–Robin spaces	– Typically occurs around the anterior commissure

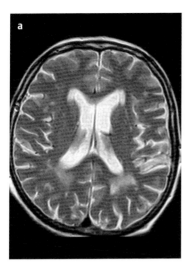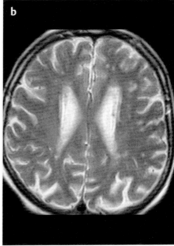

Fig. 5.7a, b Subcortical atherosclerotic encephalopathy (SAE). Axial T2-weighted MR image. Area hyperintensities in the periventricular white matter around the posterior horns of the lateral ventricles. Additional findings include multiple bilateral sharply demarcated hyperintensities on the T2-weighted image in the subcortical white matter, radiologic correlates of lacunar lesions (**a, b**).

Tips and Pitfalls

Examiners who fail to consider the ADC map can misinterpret microangiopathic changes as acute infarctions due to the T2 "shine-through" effect, which produces increased signal intensities on diffusion-weighted images.

Selected References

de Leeuw FE et al. Prevalence of cerebral white matter lesions in elderly people: a population based magnetic resonance imaging study. The Rotterdam Scan Study. J Neurol Neurosurg Psychiatry 2001; 70 (1): 9–14

Englund E. Neuropathology of white matter lesions in vascular cognitive impairment. Cerebrovasc Dis 2002; 13 (Suppl 2): 11–15

Pantoni L. Pathophysiology of age-related cerebral white matter changes. Cerebrovasc Dis 2002; 13 (Suppl 2): 7–10

Definition

▶ **Epidemiology**
Frequency: approximately 15% of all strokes.
▶ **Etiology, pathophysiology, pathogenesis**
Common causes: Hypertension ● Aneurysm ● Vascular malformation ● Tumor ●
Infarction ● Amyloid angiopathy ● Coagulation disorder.
Rare causes: Venous stasis ● Vasculitis ● Eclampsia.
Localization and etiology:
– Hematoma in basal ganglia, thalamus, pons: probably hypertensive hemor-
rhage.
– Subarachnoid hemorrhage in addition to parenchymal hemorrhage: aneu-
rysm should be considered.
– Hematoma at a different, atypical site (lobular hemorrhage): suspicion of tu-
mor, vascular malformation, dural fistula, infarction, or amyloid angiopathy.

Imaging Signs

▶ **Modality of choice**
Acute hemorrhage: CT ● Subacute and chronic hemorrhage: MRI.
▶ **CT findings**
Density on CT is determined practically exclusively by the hematocrit of the
hematoma:
– Acute hemorrhage: Hyperdensity of 150–250 HU with mass effect ● Density
decreases by approximately 1.5 HU per day.
– Hyperacute hemorrhage: Hypodensity because blood clot has not yet been ab-
sorbed ● Perifocal hypodensity (vasogenic edema) ● Ring enhancement after
two days.
▶ **MRI findings**
Signal depends on the stage of the hemorrhage and the MRI sequence (see ta-
ble) ● Ring enhancement begins after two days.
▶ **DSA**
Demonstrates the cause of the hemorrhage (such as pial or dural vascular malformation or aneurysm).

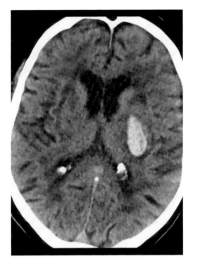

Fig. 5.8 Primary intracerebral bleeding. Axial CT. Oval hyperdensity in the left lenticular nucleus. Area hypodensities in the periventricular medulla consistent with cerebral microangiopathy.

Stage of hemorrhage	Signal in comparison with white matter		
	T1-weighted images	T2-weighted images	T2*-weighted images
Acute stage (0–24 hours) Intracellular oxyhemoglobin	Isointense	Slightly hyperintense	Slightly hypointense
Acute stage (1–3 days) Intracellular deoxyhemoglobin	Slightly hypointense	Markedly hypointense	Hypointense
Early subacute stage (3–7 days) Intracellular methemoglobin	Markedly hyperintense	Markedly hypointense	Hypointense
Late subacute stage (7–14 days) Extracellular methemoglobin	Markedly hyperintense	Markedly hyperintense	Hypointense
Chronic stage (after 14 days) Extracellular hemochromogen in the center	Isointense	Slightly hyperintense	Hypointense
Intracellular hemosiderin on the periphery	Slightly hypointense	Markedly hypointense	Markedly hypointense

Clinical Aspects

▶ **Typical presentation**
Focal neurologic deficit of acute onset according to the site of the hemorrhage •
Subarachnoid hemorrhage is associated with headache • Consciousness may be impaired.

▶ **Treatment options**
Neurosurgical decompression may be indicated depending on mass effect.

▶ **Course and prognosis**
Mortality is as high as 50% in the first few months.

▶ **What does the clinician want to know?**
Localization and cause of the hemorrhage • Follow-up • Presence of hydro-cephalus where hemorrhage enters the ventricles.

Differential Diagnosis

Ring-enhancing brain tumor   – Repeat MRI after approximately 2–6 months

Tips and Pitfalls

Failing to obtain follow-up MRI with lobular hemorrhage of unknown etiology •
Failing to obtain T2*-weighted images to demonstrate hemorrhage due to congo-philic angiopathy for Congo red dye.

Selected References

Bradley WG jr. MR appearance of hemorrhage in the brain. Radiology 1993; 189 (1): 15–26

Good CD et al. Amyloid angiopathy causing widespread miliary haemorrhages within the brain evident on MRI. Neuroradiology 1998; 40 (5): 308–311

Wakai S et al. Lobar intracerebral hemorrhage. A clinical, radiographic, and pathological study of 29 consecutive operated cases with negative angiography. J Neurosurg 1992; 76 (2): 231–238

Definition

Etiology, pathophysiology, pathogenesis
The most common cause of recurrent intracerebral hemorrhage in nonhypertensive older patients • Deposits of amyloid proteins in cortical and leptomeningeal blood vessels, cerebral cortex, and leptomeninges • The most common form is caused by the noncontractile β-amyloid protein, which displaces the contractile elements originally present in the vascular wall • It is associated to some extent with Alzheimer dementia.

Imaging Signs

▶ **Modality of choice**
MRI.

▶ **CT findings**
Confluent area hyperdensities in the subcortical and periventricular white matter consistent with vascular encephalopathy • Lobar hemorrhages are well visualized • Microhemorrhages, especially chronic ones, are usually not detectable.

▶ **MRI findings**
Confluent area hyperintensities (on T2-weighted and proton density images) or hypointensities (on T1-weighted images) in the subcortical periventricular white matter consistent with vascular encephalopathy • Lobar hemorrhage whose signal depends on the stage of the lesion • Thirty percent of patients show residues of early hemorrhages with a signal void; these are best visualized on T2*-weighted images.

Clinical Aspects

▶ **Typical presentation/Course and prognosis**
As for other intracerebral hemorrhages • Forty percent of patients exhibit subacute dementia • Fifty percent of patients develop new microhemorrhages within five years.

▶ **Treatment options**
Treatment of intracerebral hemorrhage is symptomatic • Neurosurgical decompression may be indicated.

▶ **What does the clinician want to know?**
Exclude other causes of hemorrhage • Demonstrate microhemorrhage.

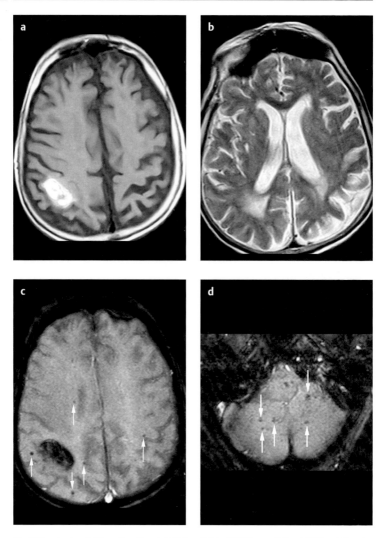

Fig. 5.9 a–d Amyloid angiopathy. Axial T1-weighted MR image (**a**), axial T2-weighted MR image (**b**), and axial T2*-weighted MR images (**c, d**). Right parietooccipital lobar hemorrhage in the extracellular methemoglobin stage (**a**). Coalescent patchy hyperintensities in the periventricular white matter representing vascular encephalopathy. Multiple signal voids a few millimeters in size (**c, d**; arrows) in the deep and subcortical white matter including the pons, radiologic correlates of chronic microhemorrhages.

Differential Diagnosis

Hypertensive hemorrhage	– Usually not multiple
	– Usually in the basal ganglia, thalamus, pons, or in the cerebellum but not at the corticomedullary junction (subcortical white matter)
Cavernous hemangiomas	– Differential diagnosis is often difficult
	– Cavernous hemangiomas occasionally enhance

Tips and Pitfalls

T2*-weighted MR images should invariably be obtained in the presence of hemorrhage of uncertain etiology and vascular encephalopathy.

Selected References

Greenberg SM. Cerebral amyloid angiopathy: prospects for clinical diagnosis and treatment. Neurology 1998; 51 (3): 690–694

Reith W. Die spontane intrazerebrale Blutung aus klinisch-neuroradiologischer Sicht. Radiologe 1999; 39 (10): 828–837

Revesz T et al. Cerebral amyloid angiopathies: a pathologic, biochemical, and genetic view. J Neuropathol Exp Neurol 2003; 62 (9): 885–898

Definition

▶ **Epidemiology**
Incidence of spontaneous dissection of the internal carotid artery is 2–3:100 000; that of dissection of the vertebral artery is 1–2:100 000 • *Peak age:* 40–50 years • Men and women are equally affected • Thirty percent of all ischemic strokes occur in young adults.

▶ **Etiology, pathophysiology, pathogenesis**
Pathogenesis: Intimal tear resulting in a false lumen and bleeding into the arterial wall • Subintimal dissection leads to stenosis; subadventitial dissection leads to aneurysmal expansion of the artery (dissecting aneurysm) • A double intimal tear can produce a false lumen that reenters the physiologic lumen.
Risk factors: Trauma • Cervical manipulations in chiropractic maneuvers • Vasculopathies such as Marfan syndrome, type IV Ehlers–Danlos syndrome, autosomal dominant polycystic kidney disorder, fibromuscular dysplasia, type I osteogenesis imperfecta.
Typical localizations:
– Extracranial internal carotid artery: from 2 cm distal to the extracranial bifurcation of the carotid to a point before the entry of the internal carotid artery into the petrous bone • In skull base fractures, dissection may also occur in the petrous or cavernous segment of the internal carotid artery.
– Extracranial vertebral artery: at the level of vertebrae C1–C2 • Rarely, in the proximal vertebral artery before its entry into the intervertebral foramen of vertebra C6.
– Middle cerebral and basilar arteries: dissections are rare.

Imaging Signs

▶ **Modality of choice**
MRI, DSA.

▶ **CT findings**
Plain CT: Usually normal.
Contrast-enhanced CT or CT angiography: Physiologic lumen enhances • False lumen can be demarcated as an intramural hematoma by the hypodense intima ("intimal flap").

▶ **MRI findings**
Depending on its age, the intramural hematoma appears isointense (acute hematoma) or hyperintense (subacute hematoma) on T1- and T2-weighted images • It is visualized even better on fat-suppressed T1-weighted images • The relationship between the intramural hematoma and the physiologic lumen is best visualized on MR angiography source images.

▶ **DSA findings**
Irregular narrowing of the artery at typical sites • Tapered stenosis in an otherwise normal vascular contour • A double lumen or intimal flap is demonstrated in less than 10% of cases.

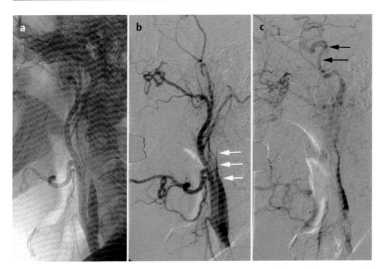

Fig. 5.10 a–c Dissection of the left internal carotid artery. Lateral DSA after injection of the left common carotid artery. Images before subtraction (**a**) and after subtraction (**b, c**). Tapered stenosis and irregularities of the wall of the cervical portion of the left internal carotid artery (**b**, white arrows). Delayed filling of the intracranial portion of the internal carotid artery (**c**, black arrows).

Clinical Aspects

▸ **Typical presentation**
Dissection of the internal carotid artery: Unilateral neck, head, facial, or orbital pain • Cranial nerve palsies involving primarily the facial, oculomotor, trigeminal, and facial nerves • Cerebral or retinal ischemia in 50–95% of cases • Oculosympathic palsy (ptosis and miosis) only occurs in less than 50% of cases.
Dissection of the vertebral artery: Neck pain and headache • Ischemia in the posterior intracranial circulatory system, in 90% of cases in the lateral medulla oblongata (Wallenberg syndrome) • Less often ischemia in the thalamus, pons, and spinal cord.

▸ **Treatment options**
Heparin in the acute phase • Later, treatment may continue with platelet aggregation inhibitors or phenprocoumon.

▸ **Course and prognosis**
This depends on the initial damage (brain infarction).

▸ **What does the clinician want to know?**
Localization and extent of the dissection • Intramural hematoma • Stenosis • Course.

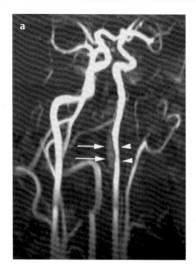 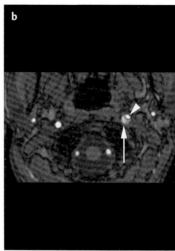

Fig. 5.11 a, b MIP reconstruction from MR angiogram (**a**) and source image from MR angiogram (**b**). Irregularities of the wall (**a**) and reduction in caliber (**a, b**) in the cervical portion of the left internal carotid artery (arrowheads). Hyperintense intramural hematoma (arrows).

Differential Diagnosis

Fibromuscular dysplasia without dissection	– Irregularly demarcated stenoses and distension of both carotid arteries at short intervals over a length of 3–5 cm at the level of vertebrae C2 and C3 – The affected segment is further proximal to these vascular segments
Thrombosis	– No intimal flap – No hematoma of the vascular wall
Arteriosclerosis	– Calcifications of the vascular wall – Changes are also intracranial and in other regions of the body
Catheter-induced vasospasm	– Spontaneously reversible within minutes

Selected References

Fiebach J et al. MRT mit Fettsuppression zur Darstellung des Wandhämatoms bei spontaner Dissektion der A. carotis interna. Röfo Fortschr Geb Röntgenstr Neuen Bildgeb Verfahr 1999; 171 (4): 290–293

Schievink WI. Spontaneous dissection of the carotid and vertebral arteries. N Engl J Med 2001; 344 (12): 898–906

Definition

▶ **Etiology, pathophysiology, pathogenesis**
Occurs in 1% of all strokes • Common predisposing factors: pregnancy, intracranial infection, desiccation, hormone therapy, coagulation disorders, tumors, trauma • Localization in order of decreasing frequency: superior sagittal sinus, transverse sinus, sigmoid sinus, cavernous sinus, internal cerebral veins • Internal cerebral venous thrombosis can lead to bilateral infarctions of basal ganglia, thalamus, hypothalamus, corpus callosum, and cerebellum.

Imaging Signs

▶ **Modality of choice**
MRI.

▶ **CT findings**
Hypodensity (vasogenic edema), possibly accompanied by parenchymal (petechial) or subarachnoid hemorrhages in the area drained by the obstructed sinus • Thrombosed sinus is hyperdense • After contrast administration, the occluded sinus appears hypodense with enhancement in the wall of the sinus (enhanced collateral veins and sinus wall produce a typical "empty triangle sign" that is detectable in 20–50% of cases).

▶ **MRI findings**
Hyperintensity on T2-and diffusion-weighted images, usually with a central area of reduced ADC • The reduced ADC returns to normal after about four days.
 – Stage I (acute thrombosis, first to fifth day): Thrombus is hypointense on T2-weighted images and isointense on proton density and T1-weighted images • The normal flow void is absent in the affected sinus.
 – Stage II (subacute thrombosis, sixth to fifteenth day): Thrombus is hyperintense on T2-weighted, proton density, and T1-weighted images.
 – Stage III (second to third week): Thrombus is hypointense on T2-weighted, proton density, and T1-weighted images.
 – Chronic stage (months): Inhomogeneous signal in the sinus (restored flow and residual thrombus).

▶ **DSA findings**
Today DSA is performed almost exclusively in the setting of local thrombolysis • Sinus lumen fails to fill • Typical venous collateralization enhances.

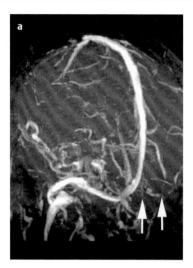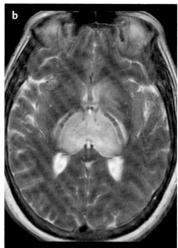

Fig. 5.12 a, b   Venous drainage impaired by extensive thrombosis. Sagittal oblique MIP reconstruction of venous MR angiogram (**a**) and axial T2-weighted MR image (**b**). Flow is obstructed by thrombosis of the internal cerebral veins, left transverse sinus (arrows), left sigmoid sinus, and left jugular vein (**a**). Bilateral edema in the thalamus (**b**).

Clinical Aspects

▶ **Typical presentation**
   Focal neurologic deficits ● Headache in 74–90% of cases ● Convulsions ● Impaired consciousness ● Optic disk edema ● Impaired vision.
▶ **Treatment options**
   Massive heparinization to increase partial thromboplastin time ● Local thrombolysis where indicated ● Symptomatic treatment of intracranial pressure ● Antiepileptic therapy ● Phenprocoumon for long-term thrombosis prophylaxis.
▶ **Course and prognosis**
   Prognosis is poor for internal cerebral venous thrombosis.
▶ **What does the clinician want to know?**
   Extent of the thrombosis ● Venous infarctions.

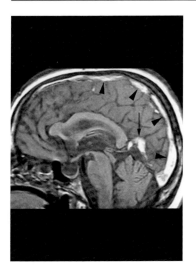

Fig. 5.13 Sagittal non-contrast-enhanced T1-weighted MR image. Subacute thrombosis of the superior sagittal sinus (arrowheads), straight sinus, and great cerebral vein of Galen (arrow) with hyperintense signal in the thrombus.

Differential Diagnosis

Arterial brain infarction	– Distribution pattern corresponds to one or several arterial territories – In the acute stage, ADC is invariably reduced in the entire infarcted area – Reduced ADC only normalizes on about the ninth day
Pseudo empty triangle sign on non-contrast-enhanced CT in a subdural hematoma or high division of the superior sagittal sinus	– Venous CT angiography and exclusion of thrombosis
Unilateral aplastic or hypoplastic transverse sinus	– In complete or partial thrombosis of the transverse sinus, a stublike part of the sinus usually fills to just distal of the confluence of the sinuses – In aplasia of the transverse sinus, there is no filling of the transverse sinus distal to the confluence of the sinuses – No abnormal venous collateralization
Pacchionian granulations that cause filling defects in the sinus	– No central filling defect but external "denting" of the sinus – Pacchionian granulations on CT have the same density as CSF, not the density of thrombus

Fig. 5.14 Coronal T1-weighted MR image after contrast administration. Thrombosis of the left sigmoid sinus with contrast void (arrow).

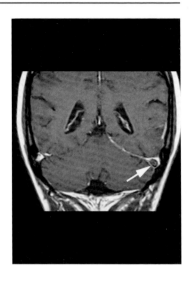

Tips and Pitfalls

Misinterpreting a unilateral aplastic or hypoplastic transverse sinus as thrombosis • Misinterpreting bilateral thalamic edema due to venous congestion as a brain tumor.

Selected References

Isensee C et al. Magnetic resonance imaging of thrombosed dural sinuses. Stroke 1994; 25 (1): 29–34

Lovblad KO et al. Diffusion-weighted MRI suggests the coexistence of cytotoxic and vasogenic oedema in a case of deep cerebral venous thrombosis. Neuroradiology 2000; 42 (10): 728–731

Renowden S. Cerebral venous sinus thrombosis. Eur Radiol 2003; 3: 3

Thron A et al. Superior sagittal sinus thrombosis: neuroradiological evaluation and clinical findings. J Neurol 1986; 233 (5): 283–288

Definition

▶ **Etiology, pathophysiology, pathogenesis**
The cause is usually circulatory collapse due to heart attack or sepsis ● Acute phase is characterized by cytotoxic cerebral edema ● Subacute stage involves reperfusion and cytotoxic and vasogenic cerebral edema ● Chronic stage involves cell death, necrosis, or gliosis ● Gray matter is selectively vulnerable ● Less severe hypoxic conditions can occur, such as altitude illness.

Imaging Signs

▶ **Modality of choice**
MRI.

▶ **CT findings**
Diffuse lesion with mass effect with bilateral obliteration of the superficial CSF spaces and narrowing of the ventricles and basal cisterns ● Basal ganglia are isodense or hypodense to white matter ● There is loss of demarcation of the cerebral cortex, initially along the border between the territories of the anterior, middle, and posterior cerebral arteries (watershed area) ● There may be a linear hyperdensity in the cerebral cortex (laminar necrosis with hemorrhages) ● The gray matter (basal ganglia, cerebral cortex) may enhance ● After a period of days to weeks, there is a decrease in the volume of the gray and white matter.

▶ **MRI findings**
  – Acute stage (< 24 hours): Swelling of the brain ● Hyperintensity (on T2-weighted, proton density, and FLAIR images) in the basal ganglia ● ADC is reduced in the cerebral cortex, basal ganglia, and cerebellum.
  – Early subacute stage (1–13 days): Hyperintensity (on T2-weighted, proton density, and FLAIR images) in the basal ganglia, cerebral cortex, and cerebellum ● ADC is reduced in the cerebral cortex and basal ganglia.
  – Late subacute stage (14–20 days): T2-weighted and T1-weighted images appear normal ● ADC is reduced in the white matter.
  – Chronic stage (> 21 days): Hyperintensity (on T2-weighted, proton density, and FLAIR images) in the basal ganglia ● T1-weighted images: Linear hyperdensities in the cerebral cortex (laminar necrosis with hemorrhages) ● ADC is normal ● Brain volume is decreased.

Clinical Aspects

▶ **Typical presentation/Course and prognosis**
Headache ● Difficulty in concentration ● Impaired coordination ● Permanent damage may be expected where hypoxia persists longer than 5 minutes ● Severe protracted hypoxia usually leads to apallic syndrome with coma.

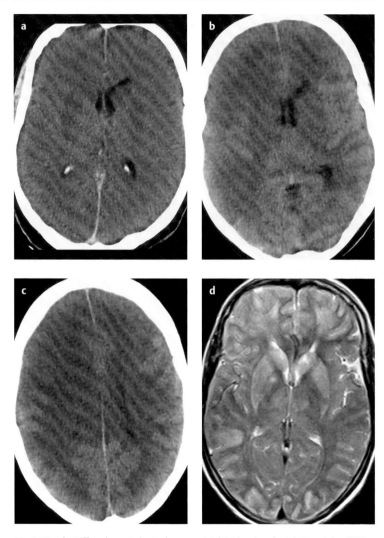

Fig. 5.15 a–d Diffuse hypoxic brain damage. Axial CT (**a–c**) and axial T2-weighted MR image (**d**). Images show total loss (**a**) or near total loss (**b, c**) of demarcation between the cerebral cortex and basal ganglia. Hyperintensity of the frontal cortex and portions of the right parietal cortex, basal ganglia, and frontal white matter (**d**).

▶ **Treatment options**
Restoration of sufficient circulatory function and respiration with oxygen ● The presence of morphologic criteria of hypoxic brain damage usually correlates with irreversible brain damage ● Then symptomatic treatment of the comatose patient is the only remaining option.

▶ **What does the clinician want to know?**
Can cerebral white matter be differentiated from cortex? ● Brain volume.

Differential Diagnosis

Hypertensive ence-phalopathy	– Changes are primarily occipital – No history of cardiac arrest
Postictal transient cerebral hyperemia	– Reversible edema
Embolic brain infarctions	– Changes occur in specific arterial territories, not diffusely throughout the entire brain

Tips and Pitfalls

Misinterpreting laminar necrosis as normal density of gray matter.

Selected References

Arbelaez A et al. Diffusion-weighted MR imaging of global cerebral anoxia. AJNR Am J Neuroradiol 1999; 20 (6): 999–1007

Han BK et al. Reversal sign on CT: effect of anoxic/ischemic cerebral injury in children. AJNR Am J Neuroradiol 1989; 10 (6): 1191–1198

Kjos BO et al. Early CT findings of global central nervous system hypoperfusion. AJR Am J Roentgenol 1983; 141 (6): 1227–1232

Tumors

Definition

▶ **Epidemiology**
Incidence in the population: 1.4% • *Sex predilection:* Females.

▶ **Etiology, pathophysiology, pathogenesis**
Slow-growing extra-axial tumor originating in the dura mater • Derived from meningothelial cells.
The histologic appearance can vary greatly:
- Meningothelial (uniform cells).
- Fibroplastic (fusiform).
- Psammomatous (irregularly calcified and ossified).
- Angiomatous (densely vascularized).
- Atypical (increased mitotic activity).
- Anaplastic malignant (sign of malignancy).

Genetics: Loss of the copy of chromosome 22. Fifteen percent of anaplastic meningiomas are associated with additional monosomies (chromosomes 10, 14, and 18) and deletion of the short arm of chromosome 1 (1 p depletion, sign of malignancy).

Imaging Signs

▶ **Modality of choice**
MRI.

▶ **CT findings**
Tumor is isodense to surrounding brain tissue • Calcifications are very common • Occasionally the entire tumor is calcified (loss of demarcation between brain tissue and skull) • Invasion and thickening (sclerosis) of the skull may occur.

▶ **Angiography findings**
Area supplied by the external carotid artery • Sphenoidal and suprasellar meningiomas may also be supplied by the internal carotid artery • "Sunrise" sign • Premature venous filling is a sign of increased vascularization or malignancy • Preoperative embolization of the tumor vessels decreases the risk of surgery.

▶ **MRI findings**
Isointense to normal brain tissue on all non-contrast-enhanced sequences • Exception: cystic meningiomas (hyperintense on T2-weighted images and hypointense on T1-weighted images) and calcified meningiomas (susceptibility artifacts) • Small meningiomas are easily missed on non-contrast-enhanced images • After contrast administration, lesions show homogeneous, significantly increased signal intensity on T1-weighted images • Broad-based meningeal attachment of the tumor: A typical sign, but one not invariably present, is the "dural tail." • With tumors located near the venous sinus, venous MR angiography or CT angiography is indicated to evaluate patency of the sinus • Infiltration of the cavernous sinus can lead to constriction of the internal carotid artery (arterial TOF angiography) • Meningiomas near the skull base can infiltrate the skull base

Tumors

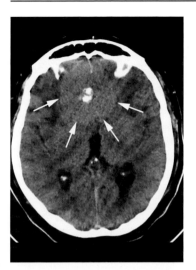

Fig. 6.1 Meningioma. Axial CT. Fronto-basal tumor slightly hyperdense to surrounding brain tissue and exhibiting central calcifications.

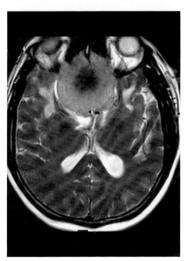

Fig. 6.2 Axial T2-weighted MR image. Frontobasal tumor slightly hyperdense to surrounding brain tissue. The central calcification is detectable because of its specific susceptibility artifact (patient from Fig. 6.**1**).

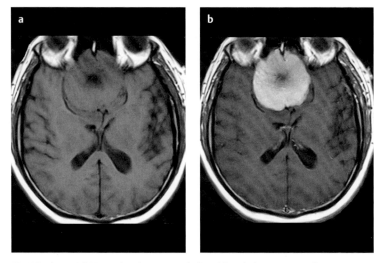

Fig. 6.3 a, b Axial T1-weighted MR image before (**a**) and after contrast administration (**b**). Tumor enhances significantly (patient from Fig. 6.1).

or the pterygopalatine fossa (via the maxillary nerve), infratemporal fossa (via the mandibular nerve), or orbits (fat-saturated T1-weighted images after contrast administration) • Infiltration of the cavernous sinus should be assumed whenever 75% of the internal carotid artery is surrounded by tumor.

Clinical Aspects

▶ **Typical presentation**
Symptoms are unspecific • Patients usually request examination because of headache or seizures • Small meningiomas are often incidental findings.
▶ **Treatment options**
Surgical resection • Radiation therapy • Somatostatin therapy.
▶ **Course and prognosis**
Prognosis is favorable where complete resection of the tumor is possible • Depending on tumor location, histology, and genetics, operable tumors may recur after surgical resection (for example where there is infiltration of the cavernous sinus) • WHO grade II tumors often recur.
▶ **What does the clinician want to know?**
Location • Size • Sinus infiltration • Vascular supply • Feasibility of arterial embolization.

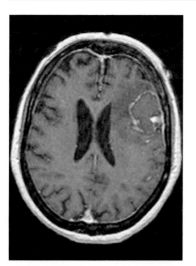

Fig. 6.4 Left frontal meningioma after intra-arterial embolization with particles. Axial T1-weighted MR image after contrast administration. The effectiveness of the embolization can be verified on MRI (only marginal enhancement).

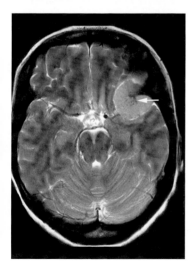

Fig. 6.5 Meningioma of the greater wing of the sphenoid. Axial T2-weighted MR image. The tumor is isointense to surrounding brain tissue. Blood vessels are visualized in the center of the tumor (flow voids, arrow).

Tumors

Fig. 6.6 Meningioma of the cerebello-pontine angle. Coronal T1-weighted MR image after contrast administration. The ring-enhancing tumor exhibits a central hypointensity consistent with calcification. The internal auditory canal (arrow) is free of tumor.

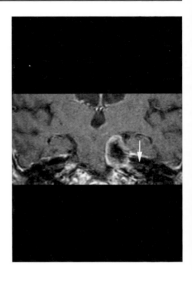

Differential Diagnosis

Hemangiopericytoma	– More rapid passage of dye and premature venous filling

Usually a differential diagnosis presents no problems as the lesion has a characteristic appearance.

Tips and Pitfalls

Failing to administer contrast and overlooking smaller meningiomas as a result.

Selected References

Grunwald I et al. Intrazerebrale Tumoren im Erwachsenenalter. Teil 2: Extraaxiale Tumoren. Radiologe 2002; 42: 840–855

Definition (WHO Grades III and IV)

▶ **Epidemiology**
Incidence: 2.6% ● *Sex predilection:* Males ● Peak age: 40–70 years.

▶ **Etiology, pathophysiology, pathogenesis**
Slightly differentiated intra-axial tumor ● Consists of pleomorphic astrocytic tumor cells with marked nuclear atypia and a significant rate of mitosis ● Pronounced microvascular proliferation ● *Histology:* Examples include anaplastic astrocytoma and oligodendroglioma, and glioblastoma ● *Genetics:* Polysomy of chromosome 7 ● Amplification of the EGFR gene consistent with heightened biological aggressiveness.

Imaging Signs

▶ **Modality of choice**
MRI.

▶ **CT findings**
Significant mass effect ● The septum pellucidum is usually displaced or the lateral ventricle compressed at the time of the diagnosis ● The center of the tumor is surrounded by a pronounced edema ● Hemorrhages consistent with malignancy are present.

▶ **MRI findings**
The tumor usually consists of a solid portion and a cystic, necrotic portion ● The center of the tumor will be isointense or hyperintense to surrounding brain tissue, depending on its cell density ● The perifocal edema is hypointense on T1-weighted images and hyperintense on T2-weighted and FLAIR images ● The edema can extend beyond the corpus callosum to the contralateral side; this is a sign of malignancy ● Solid portions of the tumor have high signal intensity on diffusion-weighted images while necrotic portions have low signal intensity ● The rrCBV is significantly increased in comparison with normal brain tissue ● An increase in rrCBV to twice normal is a sign of malignancy ● Significant ring enhancement. Usually the enhancing margin of the tumor is adjacent to the ventricular system and/or ependyma. This is a sign of beginning meningeal spread.

Clinical Aspects

▶ **Typical presentation**
Initial manifestation is usually a seizure ● Headache ● Hemiparesis occurs rarely ● Frontal tumors can lead to personality changes.

▶ **Treatment options**
Surgery ● Radiation therapy ● Chemotherapy ● There are many experimental treatments. These include hyperthermia and magnetic field therapy, although results are still inconclusive.

Tumors

Fig. 6.7 Brain tumor in the right tempo-rooccipital region. Axial CT. The rostral portions of the tumor exhibit a garland-like internal structure. The displacement of the septum pellucidum is consistent with a regional mass effect.

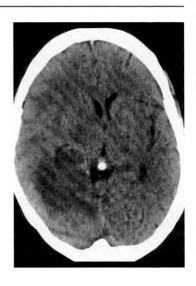

▶ **Course and prognosis**
Average survival despite maximal treatment is 14 months ● Progress has been negligible despite intensification of treatment in recent decades ● Few patients survive longer, given that complications such as wound infection secondary to craniotomy may occur.

▶ **What does the clinician want to know?**
Localization ● Size ● Grading ● Second lesion ● Ependymal or meningeal enhancement ● Obstructed CSF flow.

Differential Diagnosis

Cerebritis	– Usually lesser mass effect
	– Clinical picture with signs of inflammation
Abscess	– Greatly reduced ADC
	– Different clinical picture with signs of inflammation
Metastasis	– Ring enhancement surrounding the lesion
	– Usually located at the corticomedullary junction
	– Differential diagnosis is difficult where there is no history of primary tumor

Tips and Pitfalls

Misinterpreting an abscess as a glioblastoma.

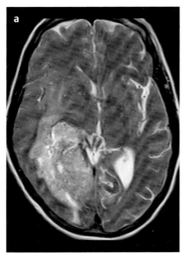

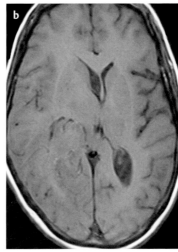

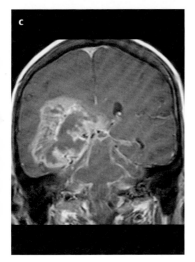

Fig. 6.8 a–c Glioblastoma. Axial T2-weighted MR image (**a**) and T1-weighted MR image (**b**) before and after (**c**) intravenous contrast administration. Inhomogeneous tumor with mass effect. The tumor enhances significantly, although meningeal perimesencephalic enhancement is seen as well (meningitis).

Fig. 6.9 Glioblastoma. Axial diffusion-weighted MR image. In addition to areas of only slightly restricted diffusion, there are also areas of significantly restricted diffusion (arrows).

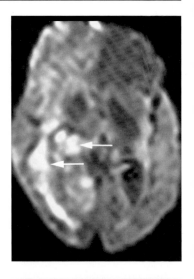

Fig. 6.10 Glioblastoma. Axial T1-weighted MR image after contrast administration. Central hypointense lesion (necrosis) surrounded by an enhancing ring (hyperintense) and a perifocal edema (hypointense).

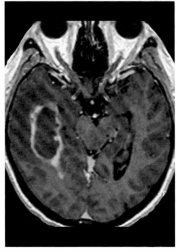

Selected References

Hartmann M et al. Funktionelle MR-Verfahren in der Diagnostik intraaxialer Hirntumoren: Perfusions- und Diffusionsbildgebung. Rofo Fortschr Geb Rontgenstr Neuen Bildgeb Verfahr 2002; 174: 955–964

Henn W et al. Genetische Grundlagen der Entstehung von Hirntumoren. Radiologe 1998; 11: 898–903

Interdisziplinäre Leitlinie der deutschen Krebsgesellschaft und ihrer Arbeitsgemeinschaften zur Diagnostik und Therapie supratentorieller Gliome des Erwachsenenalters. Onkologe 1999; 5: 831– 837

Wiestler O et al. Neuropathologie maligner Gliome. Onkologe 1998; 4: 580–588

Definition

▶ **Epidemiology**

Twenty-five percent of all brain tumors are metastases ● *Site:* 20% infratentorial, 80% supratentorial ● Peak age and sex predilection are identical to those of the primary tumor.

▶ **Etiology, pathophysiology, pathogenesis**

Secondary manifestations of an extracerebral malignant tumor ● Intracranial metastases are generally isolated, not multiple ● The most common primary tumors: Bronchial, breast, and renal cell carcinomas as well as gastrointestinal tumors and melanoma.

Imaging Signs

▶ **Modality of choice**

MRI.

▶ **CT findings**

Several processes with mass effect at various sites ● Hemorrhage will often be present (for example with melanoma metastases) ● Edema creates a perifocal hypodensity ● Larger infratentorial metastases in particular may by associated with obstructed flow of CSF or calcification (for example, with osteosarcoma metastases) ● Osteolytic or osteoblastic metastases should be evaluated in the bone window.

▶ **MRI findings**

Modality of choice for staging primary tumors (higher sensitivity than CT) ● Multiple metastases are often present ● These can occur anywhere within the central nervous system but are most commonly found at subcortical sites along the corticomedullary junction ● Lesions enhance significantly (dose dependently, with respect to both the number of metastases and the intensity of enhancement) ● Signal intensity varies with the type of primary tumor or size of the metastasis ● Melanoma metastases can be hypointense on T2-weighted images and hyperintense on T1-weighted images ● Larger metastases can exhibit central necrosis: hyperintense on T2-weighted images and hypointense on T1-weighted images ● Perfusion: significantly elevated rrCBV, but only within the margins of the tumor ● Spectroscopy: no *N*-acetylaspartate peak.

Clinical Aspects

▶ **Typical presentation**

History findings are crucial. Metastasis is suspected in patients with a known primary tumor ● Seizure ● Headache ● Vertigo ● Signs of obstructed CSF flow ● Papilledema with impaired vision.

▶ **Treatment options**

Surgical removal ● Radiation therapy ● Intrathecal cytostatic drugs.

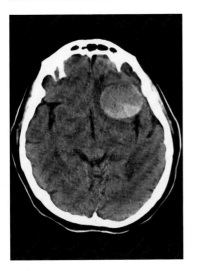

Fig. 6.11 Hemorrhaging metastasis of a malignant melanoma. Axial CT of the skull. Hyperdense tumorous lesion. Perifocal edema appears as hypodense halo. Slight midline shift to the right.

▶ **Course and prognosis**
Curative treatment is not possible where tumors metastasize to the brain • Cerebral metastasis is a late sign of malignant tumor • Patients with isolated cerebral metastases have a comparatively favorable prognosis.

▶ **What does the clinician want to know?**
Localization • Size • Multifocal?

Differential Diagnosis

Glioblastoma	– rrCBV increased even beyond the margins of the enhancing tumor – Usually unilocular
Abscess	– ADC reduced in the central necrotic area (rarely in glioblastomas and metastases as well) – rrCBV only slightly increased – Clinical and CSF findings
Pilocytic astrocytoma	– Usually younger patients – History – rrCBV only slightly increased
Hemangioblastoma	– Usually younger patients – History – rrCBV only slightly increased
Parasites	– Usually enhance less (*Echinococcus* does not enhance) – Scolex visualized

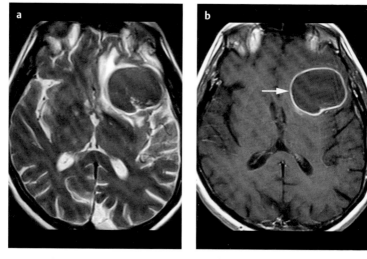

Fig. 6.12 a, b   Melanoma metastasis. Axial T2-weighted MR image (**a**) and T1-weighted MR image after contrast administration (**b**). The hypointense signal within the metastasis is consistent with a hemorrhage (deoxyhemoglobin stage). Ring enhancement (**b**, arrow; patient from Fig. **6.11**).

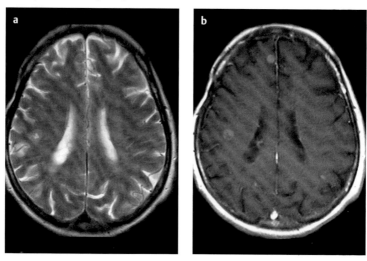

Fig. 6.13 a, b   Diffuse intracerebral metastases. Axial T2-weighted MR image (**a**) and T1-weighted MR image after contrast administration (**b**). The full extent of metastatic processes is only apparent after contrast administration.

Tips and Pitfalls

MRI not performed for staging, only cerebral CT.

Selected References

Grunwald I et al. Intrazerebrale Tumoren im Erwachsenenalter. Teil 1: Intraaxiale Tumoren. Radiologe 2002; 42: 571–587

Hartmann M et al. Funktionelle MR-Verfahren in der Diagnostik intraaxialer Hirntumoren: Perfusions- und Diffusionbildgebung. Rofo Fortschr Geb Rontgenstr Neuen Bildgeb Verfahr 2000; 174: 955–964

Definition

▶ **Epidemiology:**
Frequency: 0.15% of all brain tumors ● *Sex predilection:* Males ● *Peak age:* 50–80 years.

▶ **Etiology, pathophysiology, pathogenesis**
Intra-axial brain tumor ● Derived from astrocytes ● Diffuse astrocytomas (fibrillar, protoplasmic, and gemistocytic variants; glioblastomas) ● Tumors with a more favorable prognosis include pilocytic astrocytoma, pleomorphic xanthoastrocytoma, and subependymal giant cell astrocytoma ● Often there is a mutation of the p53 tumor suppressor gene ● Overexpression of growth gene PDGF.

Imaging Signs

▶ **Modality of choice**
MRI.

▶ **CT findings**
Hypodense in comparison with brain tissue ● Hemorrhages are rare and a sign of a higher grade tumor ● Tumor with mass effect (blurred demarcation between gray and white matter) ● There may be compression of the ventricular system and the septum pellucidum ● No enhancement.

▶ **MRI findings**
Tumor consists of several parts ● Usually there is a tumor nucleus ● The higher the cellularity of the tumor, the closer its signal will resemble gray matter ● Tumors of mild cellularity are hyperintense on T2-weighted and FLAIR images, hypointense on T1-weighted images ● A perifocal extracellular vasogenic edema of varying severity will be present ● Approximately 40% of grade II astrocytes enhance only slightly ● Lack of enhancement does not exclude a higher grade tumor ● rrCBV is similar to that of normal brain tissue ● ADC may be reduced.

Clinical Aspects

▶ **Typical presentation**
Usually asymptomatic until the time of the diagnosis ● Unspecific symptoms such as headache and vertigo ● In 65% of cases a seizure is the initial symptom of the disorder (usually a grand-mal seizure) ● Often large frontal tumor ● Personality changes may occur.

▶ **Treatment options**
Surgery, radiation therapy, and, depending on the stage, chemotherapy.

▶ **Course and prognosis**
Fifty percent of cases progress to malignancy, for which the prognosis is poor.

▶ **What does the clinician want to know?**
Size of the tumor ● Extent of the mass ● Grading ● Enhancement.

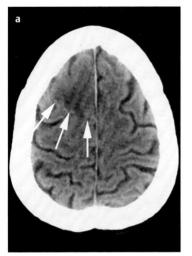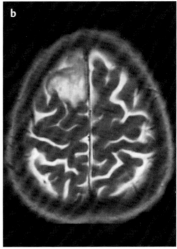

Fig. 6.14 a, b Low-grade glioma. Axial CT (**a**) and axial T2-weighted MR image (**b**). Frontal intra-axial brain tumor, hypodense on CT (**a**), hyperintense on the T2-weighted image (**b**).

Differential Diagnosis

Higher grade gliomas	– Enhancement – Usually increased diffusion
Oligodendrogliomas	– Tumor calcifications are characteristic, but they may be absent
Meningoencephalitis	– Clinical signs of infection – Abnormal CSF findings
Abscess	– ADC usually reduced in the central necrotic area – Ring enhancement
ADEM	– Typical CSF findings – Enhancement in acute stage
Multiple sclerosis	– Typical CSF findings – Clinical examination findings
Ischemia	– Usually acute onset of clinical symptoms – Seizures are very rare – Characteristic diffusion-weighted MR image – ADC reduced

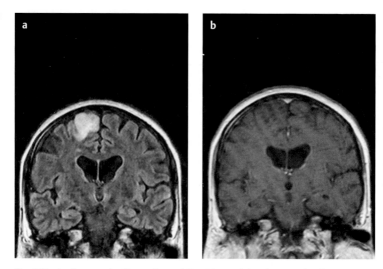

Fig. 6.15 a, b Low-grade glioma. Coronal FLAIR image (**a**) and T1-weighted MR image after contrast administration. Tumor does not enhance.

Selected References

Hartmann M et al. Funktionelle MR-Verfahren in der Diagnostik intraaxialer Hirntumoren: Perfusions- und Diffusionbildgebung. Rofo Fortschr Geb Rontgenstr Neuen Bildgeb Verfahr 2002; 174: 955–964

Henn W et al. Genetische Grundlagen der Entstehung von Hirntumoren. Radiologe 1998; 11: 898–903

Definition

▶ **Epidemiology**
Frequency: In immunocompetent persons 1.3:1 million; in immunocompromised persons 4.7:1000 ● *Sex predilection:* M:F = 2:3 ● *Peak age:* In immunocompetent persons, 50–70 years; in immunocompromised persons, below 40 years.

▶ **Etiology, pathophysiology, pathogenesis**
Malignant extranodal lymphoma without extracerebral manifestation ● Diffuse infiltration of the brain parenchyma ● Must be distinguished from cerebral lymphoma metastases in the presence of peripheral lymphomas ● *Histology:* Arranged in ring-like structures around the vessels with reticular deposits ● Distinct types include B- and T-cell lymphomas, plasmocytomas, angiotrophic lymphomas, Hodgkin lymphomas, and MALT lymphomas of the dura mater.

Imaging Signs

▶ **Modality of choice**
MRI.

▶ **CT findings**
Edema and mass effect are slight in comparison with the size of the tumor ● Tumor is hypercellular and therefore hyperdense to brain parenchyma ● Solid tumor, necrotic components are the exception (occurring in immunocompromised patients) ● Infratentorial lesions cannot be reliably diagnosed with CT.

▶ **MRI findings**
Tumor appears solid ● Rarely there are liquefied components (in immunocompromised patients) ● Isointense to normal brain tissue on the T2-weighted and T1-weighted images ● Usually homogeneously enhancing ● Involvement of the contralateral hemisphere is possible via the corpus callosum or commissures ● Multiple lesions occur in 20–40% of cases ● Due to lack of angiogenesis and the massively compromised blood–brain barrier, rrCBV is increased, although less so than with metastases and malignant gliomas ● ADC is reduced in the solid portions of the tumor.

Clinical Aspects

▶ **Typical presentation**
Unspecific symptoms ● Focal neurologic deficit (50–80% of cases) ● Neuropsychiatric symptoms (20–30% of cases) ● Papilledema (10–30% of cases) ● Ophthalmologic symptoms (such as uveitis in 5–20% of cases).

▶ **Treatment options**
Combined radiation and chemotherapy.

Tumors

Fig. 6.16 CNS lymphoma. Axial T2-weighted MR image. Hypointense tumor in the left precuneus with a significant perifocal edema.

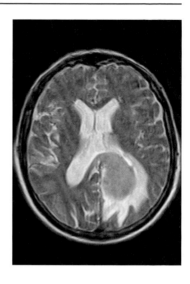

▶ **Course and prognosis**

Mean survival time is 17–45 months • Five-year survival is 25–45%.

– Favorable factors for prognosis: Unilocular • Not adjacent to CSF space • No Immunosuppression • Age below 60 years • Karnofsky index > 70.

– Unfavorable factors for prognosis: AIDS (mean survival time 13.5 months) • Angiotrophic lymphomas (rapid progression with dementia and multifocal neurologic deficit).

▶ **What does the clinician want to know?**

Localization • Size • Multiple lesions? • Diagnosis of type.

Differential Diagnosis

Glioblastoma	– Pronounced edema
	– Significant mass effect
	– Usually liquefaction and only ring enhancement
	– Radiologic differential diagnosis can be difficult in immunocompromised patients
	– CSF findings
Metastases	– Pronounced edema
	– Significant mass effect
	– History: Tumor disorder
	– CSF findings

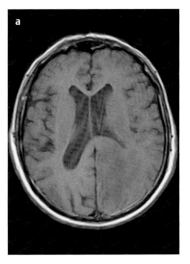 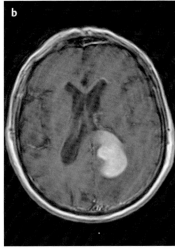

Fig. 6.17 a, b Axial T1-weighted MR image before (**a**) and after (**b**) contrast administration. Homogeneous enhancement (**b**; same case as Fig. 6.**16**).

Abscess	– Central necrotic portion with markedly restricted diffusion (hyperintense on diffusion-weighted image)
	– Invariably with liquefaction
	– CSF findings
ED	– Typical clinical picture
	– CSF findings
ADEM	– CSF findings
	– Radiologic differential diagnosis can be difficult in immunocompromised patients
Infarction	– The perfusion pattern on imaging studies can simulate a lymphoma
	– Clinical findings are typical for infarction
	– Three-week follow-up demonstrates unrestricted diffusion
	– Perfusion restriction: PTT, rrCBV, MTT

Tips and Pitfalls

Misinterpreting a necrotic lymphoma in AIDS patients as a glioblastoma.

Selected References

Feiden W et al. Primäre ZNS-Lymphome. Pathologe 2002; 23 (4): 284–291

Hartmann M et al. Funktionelle MR-Verfahren in der Diagnostik intraaxialer Hirntumoren: Perfusions- und Diffusionbildgebung. Rofo Fortschr Geb Rontgenstr Neuen Bildgeb Verfahr 2002; 174: 955–964

Herrlinger U et al. Primäre ZNS-Lymphome. Onkologe 2003; 9: 739–745

Kleihues P et al. WHO Classification of Tumours. Pathology and Genetics. Tumours of the nervous system. International Agency for Research of Cancer. Library Cataloguing in Publication Data. 2000: 129–137

Reiche W et al. Zur neuroradiologischen Diagnostik von primären Non-Hodgkin-Lymphomen des ZNS. Radiologe 1998; 38 (11): 913–923

Definition

▶ **Epidemiology**
Frequency: Pituitary adenoma 0.9%, craniopharyngioma 0.1% ● *Sex predilection:* Prolactinoma in females, craniopharyngioma in males ● *Peak age:* Pituitary adenoma after age 69 years, craniopharyngioma at age 0–10 and age 70–80 years.

▶ **Etiology, pathophysiology, pathogenesis**
These tumors arise in the sella turcica or suprasellar cisterns:
– Hormonally active and inactive adenohypophysial adenomas
– Craniopharyngioma (adamantine type: calcifications, in children; papillary type: no calcifications, in adults, derived from the epithelium of the Rathke's pouch)
– Rathke cleft cysts
– Tumors of the pituitary stalk (histiocytosis, metastases, germinomas)
– Primary tumors arising from the neurohypophysis (such as choristomas) are rare

Imaging Signs

▶ **Modality of choice**
MRI.

▶ **CT findings**
Tumor is isodense to normal brain tissue ● Lies between clinoid process and dorsum sellae ● Masks suprasellar cisterns ● Displacement of the structures of the base of the brain ● Large tumors may lead to obstructed CSF flow ● Craniopharyngiomas in children are often calcified ● Calcifications in adults are the exception ● Multiple detector systems can be used to generate sagittal and coronal reconstructions (such as in patients with cardiac pacemakers).

▶ **MRI findings**
Pituitary adenoma: Cranial displacement of the pituitary (convex margin; a certain degree of convexity may be normal in young women) ● Displacement of the pituitary stalk ● Asymmetry of the sellar floor ● Inhomogeneity on T1-weighted images ● Prolactinomas can be hyperintense to brain tissue on non-contrast-enhanced T1-weighted images, hyperintense on T2-weighted images, and hypointense on T1-weighted images after contrast administration ● Macroadenomas may include cystic components ● Microadenomas are smaller than 1 cm, macroadenomas larger than 1 cm ● Microadenomas can be so small that they are undetectable on MRI ● Infiltration of the cavernous sinus is difficult to evaluate on MRI ● Rule of thumb: where the tumor surrounds at least 75% of the circumference of the internal carotid artery, the cavernous sinus is infiltrated.
Craniopharyngioma: Primarily cystic tumor ● Signal intensity of cyst contents varies with their protein content ● Asymmetrically enhancing solid component.

Tumors

Fig. 6.18 Craniopharyngioma. Coronal T1-weighted MR image after contrast administration. Cyst contents already hyperintense on non-contrast-enhanced T1-weighted images (not shown) with thin rim of enhancement representing the cyst wall. The widening of the temporal horns of the lateral ventricles is a sign of obstructed CSF flow (blockage of the interventricular foramen of Monro by the tumor).

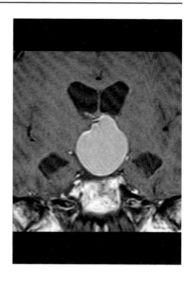

Clinical Aspects

▶ **Typical presentation**

Hormonally active adenoma: Acromegaly ● Cushing syndrome ● Galactorrhea ● Infertility ● Changes in laboratory parameters (elevated prolactin, ACTH, STH) ● These changes may be very small at the time of the initial diagnosis (microadenoma).

Other sellar tumors: Cardinal symptom is homonymous hemianopsia due to compression of the optic chiasm ● Lesions of other cranial nerves are rare.

▶ **Treatment options**

Pituitary adenoma: Medical therapy for prolactinoma ● Surgical resection, usually via sphenoidotomy ● All other types of adenoma are treated by surgical resection.

Craniopharyngioma: Surgical resection.

Rathke cleft cyst: Observation ● Surgical resection where there is compression of the optic chiasm.

Metastases, Langerhans cell histiocytosis: Radiation therapy ● Steroids.

Sarcoidosis: Steroid therapy.

▶ **Course and prognosis**

Prognosis is good where there is no infiltration of the cavernous sinus ● However, craniopharyngiomas in particular frequently recur.

▶ **What does the clinician want to know?**

Location of the adenoma ● Compression of the optic chiasm ● Infiltration of the cavernous sinus (difficult diagnosis) ● Sellar or suprasellar tumor.

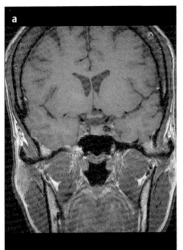

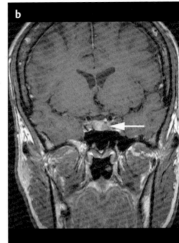

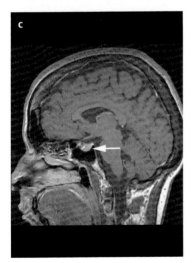

Fig. 6.19 a–c Microadenoma of the anterior pituitary lobe. Coronal T1-weighted MR image before (**a**) and after (**b**) intravenous contrast administration. Sagittal T1-weighted MR image after contrast administration (**c**). The T1-weighted image after contrast administration shows less enhancement in the microadenoma than in normal pituitary tissue (**b, c**; arrow).

Differential Diagnosis

Meningioma	– Usually relatively large extrasellar component
	– A "dural tail" has also been described in pituitary adenomas
Abscess	– Clinical and CSF findings
Metastases	– Usually multiple (e.g., breast carcinoma, melanoma)
	– Involvement of the infundibulum
	– Differential diagnosis can be difficult where larger isolated tumors are present
	– History

Tips and Pitfalls

Failing to obtain non-contrast-enhanced study ● Dispensing with thin-slice T2-weighted sequence (misinterpreting pituitary cysts).

Selected References

Cottier JP et al. Cavernous sinus invasion by pituitary adenoma: MR imaging. Radiology 2000; 215: 463–469

Hagiwara, Y et al. Comparison of growth hormone-producing and non-growth hormone-producing pituitary adenomas: Imaging characteristics and pathologic correlation. Radiology, 2003; 228 (2): 533–538

Karnaze MG et al. Suprasellar lesions: evaluation with MR imaging. Radiology 1986; 161: 77–82

Kobayashi S et al. A clinical and histopathological study of factors affecting MRI signal intensities of pituitary adenomas. Neuroradiology. 1994; 36 (4): 298–302

Definition

▶ **Epidemiology**
Frequency: Schwannoma: 8% of all intracranial tumors • Neurofibroma: no data in the literature • Malignant peripheral nerve sheath tumor: 5% of all malignant soft tissue tumors • Metastases: rare.
Sex predilection: Schwannoma: M:F = 1:2 • Neurofibroma: no sex predilection • Malignant peripheral nerve sheath tumor: no sex predilection • Metastases: no sex predilection.
Peak age: Schwannoma: 30–60 years • Neurofibroma: no peak age. Malignant peripheral nerve sheath tumor: 20–50 years • Metastases: 30–80 years.

▶ **Etiology, pathophysiology, pathogenesis**
Tumors derived from the sheaths of the cranial nerves • Neural tumors are classified as either schwannomas (fusiform Schwann cells, hypocellular) or neurofibromas (type I neurofibromatosis, hypercellular, mixture of Schwann cells and fibroblasts) • With secondary nerve sheath tumors, a distinction is made between metastases and malignant nerve sheath tumor.

Imaging Signs

▶ **Modality of choice**
MRI.

▶ **CT findings**
CT can confirm the diagnosis only where there are extensive findings • CT usually fails to detect intrameatal vestibular nerve tumors or foraminal trigeminal neurinomas • Isodense tumor • Obstructed CSF flow • Calcifications are rare • Large tumors are associated with widened foramina and bony destruction (for example, foramen ovale, foramen rotundum, and internal auditory canal).

▶ **MRI findings**
Neural tumors on non-contrast-enhanced images are usually isointense • Localized thickening of the nerve and pronounced enhancement (homogeneous with neurinomas and schwannomas, inhomogeneous with malignant tumor proliferation and metastases) • Cystic neurinomas are hypointense to brain tissue on T1-weighted images and hyperintense on T2-weighted images • One contrast sequence must be fat saturated (customarily the coronal sequence) • The T2-weighted sequence must be at high resolution with a voxel size less than 1 mm^3.

Clinical Aspects

▶ **Typical presentation**
Pain is usually a sign of a malignant tumor.
Neurologic impairment:
  – Vestibular neurinoma: hearing impairment, facial paresis.
  – Trigeminal neurinoma: unilateral facial hypesthesia; pain is rare.
  – Glossopharyngeal neurinoma: difficulty swallowing.

Fig. 6.20 Vestibular neurinoma. Axial CT. Widening of the internal auditory canal and destruction of the posterior bony margin are indirect signs of a large vestibular neurinoma.

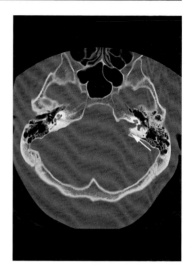

▶ **Treatment options**

Neurinomas and schwannomas are treated by surgical resection ● Radiation therapy (gamma knife) where indicated ● Metastases and malignant peripheral nerve sheath tumors are irradiated.

▶ **Course and prognosis**

Prognosis is good for schwannoma and neurofibroma ● Surgical risk includes loss of nerve function (hearing loss, sensory deficits) ● Metastases and malignant peripheral nerve sheath tumors in particular are late signs of malignant disease with a poor prognosis.

▶ **What does the clinician want to know?**

Which nerve is affected? ● Does the tumor grow through the base of the skull and if it does, where? ● Extent ● Distance to endangered anatomic structures (such as the ampulla of the labyrinth).

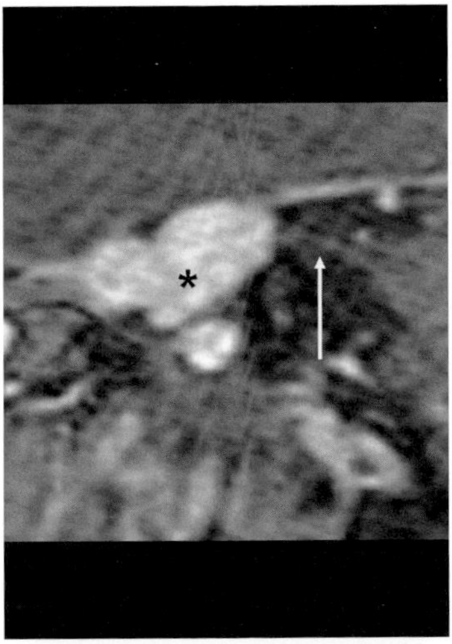

Fig. 6.21 Sagittal reconstruction from a three-dimensional T1-weighted MR sequence after contrast administration. Hourglass-shaped maxillary neurinoma (*). Homogeneous enhancement (arrow = trigeminal nerve).

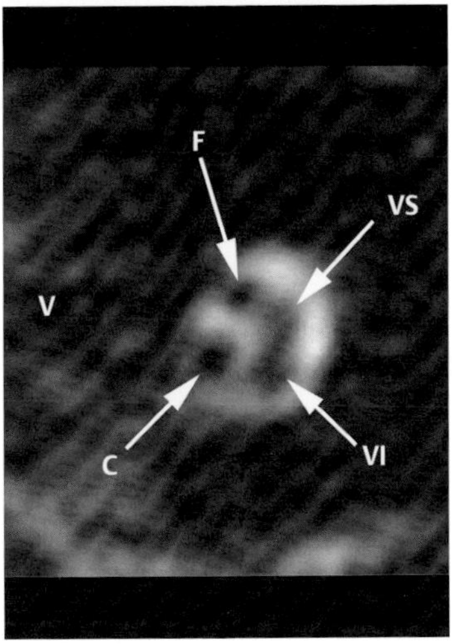

Fig. 6.22 Sagittal reconstruction through the internal auditory canal from a three-dimensional T2-weighted TRUE FISP sequence. (V = anterior (ventral); F = facial nerve; VS = superior vestibular nerve; VI = interior vestibular nerve; c = cochlear nerve.)

Tumors

Differential Diagnosis

Inflammation	– Typical brief history, often in combination with a respiratory tract infection
	– The nerve itself is not thickened
	– The lesion has ill-defined margins and enhances less than tumors
	– Enhancement persists on follow-up studies up to six months after clinical symptoms have subsided
Arachnoid cyst	– Does not enhance
	– No thickening of the nerve
Hemangioma	– Hemosiderin artifact on T2*-weighted MR images (note that many artifacts occur in this sequence near the base of the skull)
	– Hyperintense on non-contrast-enhanced T1-weighted MR images in the presence of hemorrhage
Lipoma	– Hyperintense on non-contrast-enhanced T1-weighted MR images
	– Hyperintensity disappears with fat saturation
Neurovascular impingement with neuralgia	– A blood vessel compressing the nerve can be clearly identified
	– Atrophy of the nerve

Tips and Pitfalls

No fat saturation after contrast administration.

Selected References

Blandino A et al. CT and MR findings in neoplastic perineural spread along the Vidian nerve. Europ. Radiol 2000; 10 (3): 521–526

De Foer B. Tumours of the cerebellopontine angle, internal auditory canal and inner ear. In Lemmerling M., Kollias S. Radiology of the petrous bone. Berlin, Heidelberg, New York: Springer; 2004: 130–142

Kleihues Pet al. WHO Classification of Tumours. Pathology and Genetics. Tumours of the nervous system. International Agency for Research of Cancer. Library Cataloguing in Publication Data. 2000: 129–137

Williams LS. Advanced concepts in the imaging of perineural spread of tumor to the trigeminal nerve. Top Magn Reson Imaging 1999; 10 (6): 376–383

Definition

▶ **Epidemiology**

Frequency: 0.29% of all intracranial tumors ● *Sex predilection:* Males ● *Peak age:* 20–70 years.

▶ **Etiology, pathophysiology, pathogenesis**

Medium cellular density ● Derived from oligodendrocytes ● Honeycomb structure in histologic specimen with microcalcifications ● Dense capillary network ● Loss of chromosome 10 with astrocytic component ● Loss of the short arm of chromosome 1 is specific for the oligodendrocytic component.

Imaging Signs

▶ **Modality of choice**

MRI.

▶ **CT findings**

Calcifications are characteristic (50% of all lesions) ● However, absence of calcifications does not exclude oligodendroglioma ● Mass effect ● Hypodense with perifocal edema.

▶ **MRI findings**

Susceptibility artifacts (calcifications) ● Tumor center: The higher the cellularity of the tumor, the more the tumor will be isointense to brain tissue on all sequences ● Tumors of mild cellularity are hyperintense on T2-weighted and FLAIR images and hypointense to brain tissue on T1-weighted images ● Perifocal extracellular edema of varying severity will be present ● Cystic lesions ● Significantly increased rrCBV in grade II oligodendrogliomas (very dense capillary network).

Clinical Aspects

▶ **Typical presentation**

Usually asymptomatic until the time of the diagnosis ● Unspecific symptoms such as headache and vertigo ● In 65% of cases, a seizure is the initial symptom of the disorder (usually a grand-mal seizure) ● Frontal tumors may already be quite large (sole symptom is personality changes).

▶ **Treatment options**

Surgical removal ● Radiation therapy ● Chemotherapy where indicated.

▶ **Course and prognosis**

Fifty percent of all cases progress to malignancy, for which the prognosis is poor.

▶ **What does the clinician want to know?**

Localization ● Extent ● Obstructed CSF flow ● Diagnosis of type if possible.

Fig. 6.23 Oligodendroglioma. Axial CT. Tumor with typical coarse calcifications and pronounced perifocal edema.

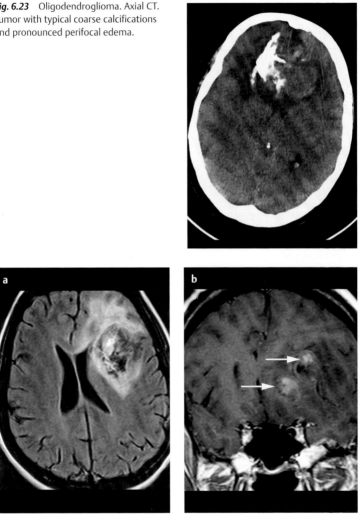

Fig. 6.24a, b Oligodendroglioma. Axial FLAIR image (**a**) and coronal T1-weighted MR image after contrast administration (**b**). Perifocal edema and susceptibility artifact (hypointense) consistent with calcification (**a**). Enhancement (arrows) may occur even in low-grade oligodendrogliomas (**b**; increased capillary density and not a sign of compromised blood-brain barrier).

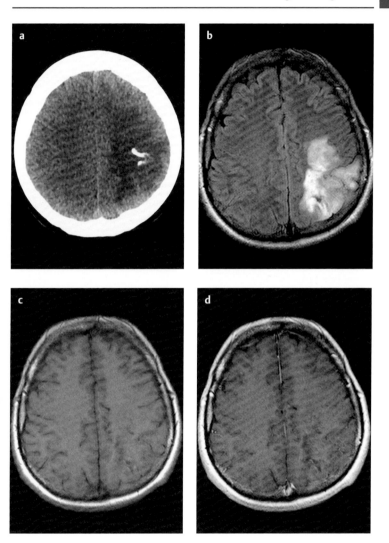

Fig. 6.25 a–d Oligodendroglioma. Axial CT (**a**), FLAIR (**b**), T1-weighted non-contrast-enhanced (**c**) and contrast-enhanced MR images (**d**). Left parietal oligodendroglioma with central calcification. This WHO grade II tumor does not enhance.

Differential Diagnosis

Glioblastoma	– Clinical course
	– Necrosis
	– Significant enhancement
Anaplastic oligo-dendroglioma	– Clinical course
	– Differential diagnosis based solely on imaging findings can be difficult
Dysembryoplastic neuro-epithelial tumor (DNT)	– Only slight perifocal edema or none at all
	– Localization: temporal lobe

Tips and Pitfalls

Excluding an oligodendroglioma because of the absence of calcifications.

Selected References

Grunwald I et al. Intrazerebrale Tumoren im Erwachsenenalter. Teil 1: Intraaxiale Tumoren. Radiologe 2002; 42: 571–587

Hartmann M et al. Funktionelle MR-Verfahren in der Diagnostik intraaxialer Hirntumoren: Perfusions- und Diffusionbildgebung. Rofo Fortschr Geb Rontgenstr Neuen Bildgeb Verfahr 2002; 174: 955–964

Definition

▸ **Epidemiology**
Frequency: 0.3% of all intracranial tumors ● *Sex predilection:* Males ● *Peak age:* 0–20 years.

▸ **Etiology, pathophysiology, pathogenesis**
Hypocellular intra-axial tumor derived from astrocytes ● Low rate of mitosis ● Common site: infratentorial (cerebellum, pons) ● Supratentorial lesions are usually in the region of the third ventricle or superior to the optic chiasm.

Imaging Signs

▸ **Modality of choice**
MRI

▸ **CT findings**
Cystic (hypodense) and solid (isodense) tumor components ● Calcifications may occur ● Infratentorial lesions can compress the fourth ventricle and aqueduct of Sylvius, obstructing the flow of CSF (widening of the temporal horns of the lateral ventricles) ● Hemorrhages are rare.

▸ **MRI findings**
Lesion with mass effect ● Only slight perifocal edema ● T1-weighted image: cyst hypointense to white matter and isointense solid tumor component ● T2-weighted image: hyperintense cyst and isointense solid tumor component ● FLAIR image: hypointense cyst and hyperintense solid tumor component ● T1-weighted image after contrast administration: pronounced asymmetrical enhancement.

Clinical Aspects

▸ **Typical presentation**
Signs of elevated intracranial pressure: Vomiting (especially on an empty stomach) ● Headache ● Failure to thrive ● Retarded development ● Increase in cranial circumference ● Stiff neck.
Functional impairments of the caudal brainstem: Abducent nerve palsy ● Impaired consciousness.
Cerebral symptoms: Palsies ● Seizures ● Impaired visual acuity ● Personality changes ● Impaired speech.
Suprasellar location: Limited visual acuity and visual field defects ● Endocrine dysfunction ● Diencephalic syndrome ● Palsies ● Reversal of sleep–wake rhythm.
Location in posterior cranial fossa and brainstem: Ataxia ● Nystagmus ● Intention tremor ● Deficits in long pathways ● Dysregulation of vital centers ● Cranial nerve deficits.

▸ **Treatment options**
Surgical removal ● Radiation therapy where indicated.

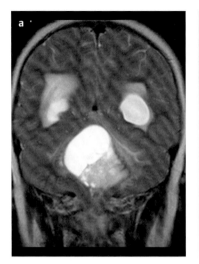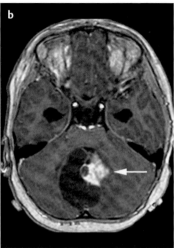

Fig. 6.26 a, b Pilocytic astrocytoma of the cerebellum. Coronal T2-weighted MR image (**a**) and axial T1-weighted MR image after contrast administration (**b**). Cystic component of the tumor appears hyperintense on the T2-weighted image and hypointense on the T1-weighted image. Solid tumor component enhances (arrow).

▸ **Course and prognosis**
  Prognosis is good; 10-year survival is about 78%.
▸ **What does the clinician want to know?**
  Localization ● Extent ● Differential diagnosis to exclude hemangioblastoma and glioblastoma.

Differential Diagnosis

Hemangioblastoma	– Similar appearance on CT and MRI
	– Pilocytic astrocytoma usually occurs in children, whereas hemangioblastoma usually occurs in adults
Medulloblastoma	– Similar peak age and common site
	– Usually lacking cystic components on MRI
	– Enhancement usually not very pronounced
Ependymoma	– Similar common site
	– Different peak age
	– Different appearance on MRI
Glioblastoma	– Pronounced edema
	– Restricted diffusion
	– Increased rrCBV

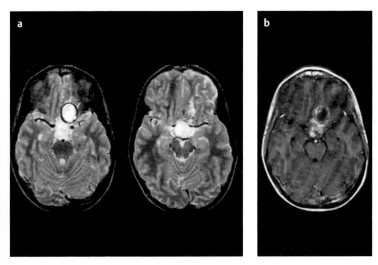

Fig. 6.27 a, b　Suprasellar pilocytic astrocytoma. Axial T2-weighted MR image (**a**) and T1-weighted MR image after contrast administration (**b**).

Metastases	– Usually not symmetrically enhancing
	– Pronounced edema
	– Rare in children
Lymphoma	– Usually no cystic component. Increased rrCBV
Plexus tumors	– Usually clearly related to the ventricular system

Tips and Pitfalls
....

Misinterpreting as glioblastoma.

Selected References

Grunwald I et al. Intrazerebrale Tumoren im Erwachsenenalter. Teil 1: Intraaxiale Tumoren. Radiologe 2002; 42: 571–587

Hartmann M et al. Funktionelle MR-Verfahren in der Diagnostik intraaxialer Hirntumoren: Perfusions- und Diffusionbildgebung. Rofo Fortschr Geb Rontgenstr Neuen Bildgeb Verfahr 2002; 174: 955–964

Henn W et al. Genetische Grundlagen der Entstehung von Hirntumoren. Radiologe 1998; 11: 898–903

Definition

► **Epidemiology**
Frequency: 0.5:100 000 children under 15 ● *Sex predilection:* Males ● *Peak age:* 0–10 years ● Seventy percent of all patients are younger than 16 years.

► **Etiology, pathophysiology, pathogenesis**
Malignant embryonal tumor of the cerebellum (primary neuroectodermal tumor) ● Drop metastases ● Histology: Densely packed round to oval cells with hyperchromatic nuclei ● Typical findings include neuroblast rosettes ● WHO grade IV ● Localization: 75% occur in the cerebellar vermis in the vicinity of the fourth ventricle ● In adults, the cerebellar hemispheres are involved (desmoplastic type).

Imaging Signs

► **Modality of choice**
MRI.

► **CT findings**
Inhomogeneous cerebellar tumor ● Hemorrhages may occur ● Calcifications are rare ● Tumor will not necessarily enhance.

► **MRI findings**
Infiltrating tumor ● Usually lies in the midline and involves the cerebellar vermis ● Inhomogeneous signal pattern ● Compression of the fourth ventricle ● Infiltration of the ventricular systems is common ● Main portion of the tumor usually lies outside the CSF space ● Compression of the brainstem (pons and cerebellar peduncles) ● Inhomogeneous enhancement ● Obstructed CSF flow ● Drop metastases may occur in the entire CSF space (these too will not necessarily enhance).

Clinical Aspects

► **Typical presentation**
Cerebellar symptoms (ataxia) ● Obstructed CSF flow (nausea, vomiting, headache).

► **Treatment options**
Surgical resection ● Combined radiation and chemotherapy.

► **Course and prognosis**
Prognosis is less favorable in patients under age 3 years, with metastases, or who received subtotal surgical resection ● Five-year survival rate is 50–70% (reflecting improvements in perioperative care, imaging, surgical technique, and radiation therapy protocols) ● Prognosis is more favorable for desmoplastic medulloblastomas, less favorable for large-cell variants of medulloblastoma.

► **What does the clinician want to know?**
Extent ● Localization ● Diagnosis of type ● Metastases ● Obstructed CSF flow.

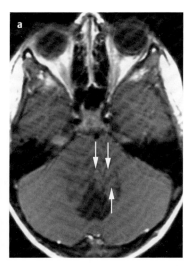 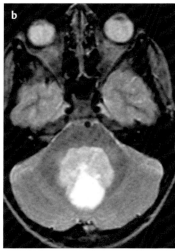

Fig. 6.28 a, b Medulloblastoma. Axial T1-weighted MR image after contrast administration (**a**) and axial T2-weighted MR image (**b**). Inhomogeneously enhancing tumor arising from the cerebellar vermis (arrows). Compression of the fourth ventricle and bilateral infiltration of the middle cerebellar peduncle.

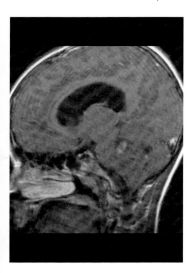

Fig. 6.29 Medulloblastoma. Sagittal T1-weighted MR image after contrast administration. Tumor is adjacent to the ventricular system and cerebellum. The pons is displaced anteriorly, the cerebellar hemispheres posteriorly, and the cerebellar tonsils into the foramen magnum. Same case as Fig. 6.**28**.

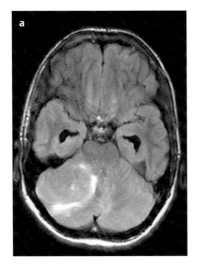

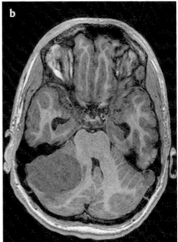

Fig. 6.30 a–c Desmoplastic medulloblastoma of the right cerebellar hemisphere. Axial FLAIR image (**a**), axial T1-weighted MR image before (**b**) and after contrast administration (**c**). Desmoplastic medulloblastomas occur primarily in adolescents and young adults.

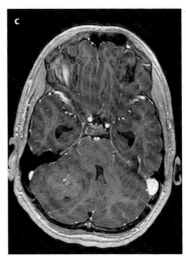

Differential Diagnosis

Ependymoma	– Significant enhancement
	– Arises from ventricular system
	– Infiltrates the cerebellum
Pilocytic astrocytoma	– Does not infiltrate the ventricular system
	– Usually part of the tumor enhances significantly
	– Cystic component
Epidermoid	– Usually lateral, not in the midline, extra-axial
	– Adjacent to subarachnoid space
	– Does not enhance
	– Greatly reduced ADC
Plexus tumors	– Arise from ventricular system
	– Significant enhancement
Hemangioblastoma	– Different age group
	– Not adjacent to ventricular system
	– Part of the tumor enhances significantly

Tips and Pitfalls

Failing to examine brain and spinal cord completely and missing metastases as a result.

Selected References

Buhring U et al. MRI features of primary, secondary and metastatic medulloblastoma. Eur Radiol. 2002; 12 (6): 1342–1348

Kleihues P et al. WHO Classification of Tumours. Pathology and Genetics. Tumours of the nervous system. International Agency for Research of Cancer. Library Cataloguing in Publication Data. 2000: 129–137

Kortmann R et al. Aktuelle und zukünftige Strategien in der interdisziplinären Therapie von Medulloblastomen, supratentoriellen PNET und intrakraniellen Keimzelltumoren im Kindesalter. Strahlentherapie und Onkologie 2001; 177 (9): 447–461

Definition

....

▶ **Epidemiology**
Incidence: Pineoblastoma: 45% of all pineal tumors ● Germinoma: 0.3% of all brain tumors ● Pineocytoma: 1% of all brain tumors.
Sex predilection: Pineoblastoma: males ● Germinoma: M:F = 2:1 ● Pineocytoma: no sex predilection.
Peak age: Pineoblastoma: 0–20 years ● Germinoma: 10–20 years ● Pineocytoma: 20–40 years.

▶ **Etiology, pathophysiology, pathogenesis**
Tumors arising from the pineal gland ● Benign tumors (pineal cyst, pineocytomas, teratoma, dermoid) are differentiated from malignant tumors (germinoma, pineoblastoma, choriocarcinoma) ● Tumors derived from pineal cells are differentiated to varying degrees depending on their malignancy ● Germinomas are derived from primitive germ cells; teratomas typically consist of ectodermal, endodermal, and mesenchymal components of varying degrees of differentiation (mature teratoma, teratocarcinoma).

Imaging Signs

....

▶ **Modality of choice**
MRI.

▶ **CT findings**
Homogeneous tumor in the pineal region superior and posterior to the quadrigeminal plate ● Calcifications can occur, especially in germinomas and pineocytomas ● Even small tumors can lead to obstructed CSF flow ● In contrast to the smooth margins of the pineocytoma, the pineoblastoma has an indistinct irregular margin ● Germinomas are hyperdense to the surrounding brain parenchyma ● Pineoblastomas and pineocytomas are hypodense.

▶ **MRI findings**
Pineocytoma: Hypointense to brain tissue on T1-weighted images, hyperintense on T2-weighted images ● Homogeneous enhancement ● Usually smaller than 3 cm.
Pineoblastoma: Hypointense on T1-weighted images, hyperintense on T2-weighted images ● Inhomogeneous enhancement ● Often larger than 3 cm ● Lobulated.
Germinoma: Solid tumor ● Significant enhancement ● Drop metastases in the CSF space.
Teratoma: Ring enhancement ● Intratumor cyst may be present ● Signal varies according to the relative content of the three types of cells.
Choriocarcinoma: Hemorrhages are characteristic ● Enhancement is seen along with necrotic areas that appear hypointense on T1-weighted images.

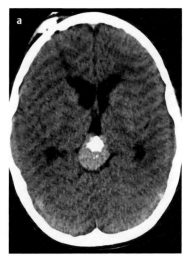
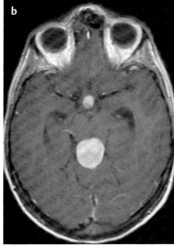

Fig. 6.31 a, b Pineal germinoma. Axial CT without (**a**) and axial T1-weighted MR image after contrast administration (**b**). CT shows a moderately hyperdense tumor with coarse, eccentric calcification (**a**). Significant enhancement (b) both in the pineal body and in the infundibular region (multilocular involvement).

Clinical Aspects

▶ **Typical presentation**
   Obstructed CSF flow: Headache ● Nausea ● Vomiting ● Vertigo ● Impaired vision with papilledema.
▶ **Treatment options**
   Treatment of the obstructed CDF flow: Shunt ● Ventriculostomy ● Irradiation.
▶ **Course and prognosis**
   Pineocytoma: Five-year survival rate: 86% ● *Pineoblastoma:* Five-year survival rate: 58% ● *Germinoma, teratoma:* Five-year survival rate: 65–95%.
▶ **What does the clinician want to know?**
   Obstructed CSF flow ● Extent of tumor ● Drop metastases.

Differential Diagnosis

Metastasis	– Often history of primary tumor
	– Can be difficult to distinguish from pineal tumor
Arachnoid cyst	– Does not enhance
	– Homogeneous structure isointense to fluid
Pilocytic astrocytoma	– Peripineal location
	– Cystic component enhances asymmetrically

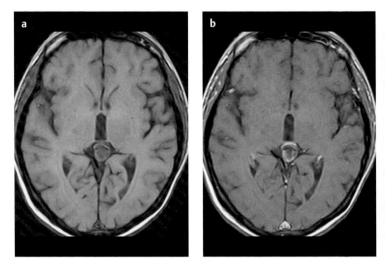

Fig. 6.32 a, b Pineocytoma. Axial T1-weighted MR image before (**a**) and after contrast administration (**b**). Hypointense tumor in the pineal region (**a**), ring enhancement.

Selected References

Kleihues P et al. WHO Classification of Tumours. Pathology and Genetics. Tumours of the nervous system. International Agency for Research of Cancer. Library Cataloguing in Publication Data. 2000: 129–137

Mader I et al. Die kernspintomographische Differentialdiagnose von Tumoren der Pinealisregion. Klinische Neuroradiologie 2001; 11 (1): 25–32

Definition

▶ **Epidemiology**
  Incidence: 1% of all intracranial tumors ● *Peak age:* 30–40 years.
▶ **Etiology, pathophysiology, pathogenesis**
  Keratin-containing epidermal tumor ● Slow-growing ● Localization: 40% occur
  in the cerebellopontine angle as extra-axial tumors.

Imaging Signs

▶ **Modality of choice**
  MRI.
▶ **CT findings**
  Hypodense tumor ● Calcifications occur in 25% of all cases ● Mass effect with
  displacement of brain structures can occur with sufficiently large tumors ● Tu-
  mors in the posterior cranial fossa can lead to obstructed CSF flow ● No enhance-
  ment ● Compression may cause regional thinning of the inner table.
▶ **MRI findings**
  Tumors are usually isointense to fluid on T2-weighted and T1-weighted im-
  ages ● Ring enhancement is rare (a sign of inflammation) ● Large tumors lead
  to obstructed CSF flow ● Tumor contents appear hyperintense on FLAIR images ●
  Diffusion-weighted images show greatly restricted diffusion.
▶ **Characteristic findings**
  Pronounced diffusion restriction.

Clinical Aspects

▶ **Typical presentation**
  Clinical symptoms of a mass: Headache ● Vertigo ● Vomiting and nausea ● Papil-
  ledema with obstructed CSF flow.
  Lesion in the cerebellopontine angle: Hearing impairment ● Facial paresis.
▶ **Treatment options**
  Surgical removal.
▶ **Course and prognosis**
  Tumor may recur ● Total resection of tumors in the cerebellopontine angle or
  prepontine tumors is usually not feasible.
▶ **What does the clinician want to know?**
  Localization ● Extent ● Diagnosis of type.

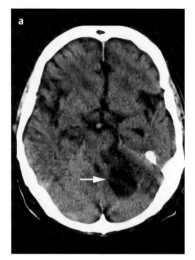

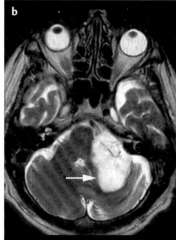

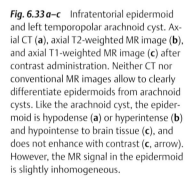

Fig. 6.33 a–c Infratentorial epidermoid and left temporopolar arachnoid cyst. Axial CT (**a**), axial T2-weighted MR image (**b**), and axial T1-weighted MR image (**c**) after contrast administration. Neither CT nor conventional MR images allow to clearly differentiate epidermoids from arachnoid cysts. Like the arachnoid cyst, the epidermoid is hypodense (**a**) or hyperintense (**b**) and hypointense to brain tissue (**c**), and does not enhance with contrast (**c**, arrow). However, the MR signal in the epidermoid is slightly inhomogeneous.

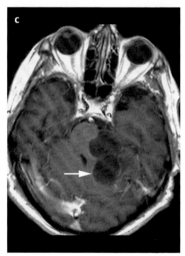

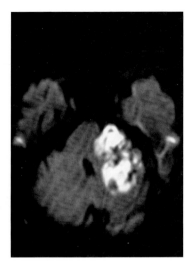

Fig. 6.34 Axial diffusion-weighted MR image (*b* = 1000). Now it is possible to distinguish an arachnoid cyst from an epidermoid. Epidermoids show a significant diffusion restriction (hyperintense), whereas arachnoid cysts facilitate diffusion (hypointense; patient from Fig. 6.**33**).

Differential Diagnosis

Arachnoid cyst	– Appearance similar to CSF on T1-weighted, T2-weighted, FLAIR, and diffusion-weighted MR images (ADC not reduced relative to CSF) – Smooth margin
Lipoma	– Hyperintense on T1-weighted MR images – Fat suppression eliminates the hyperintense signal
Dermoid	– Contains other components from epidermal tissue development (hair, teeth) – Hyperintense on T1-weighted MR images

Tips and Pitfalls

Misinterpreting as an arachnoid cyst.

Selected References

Grunwald I et al. Intrazerebrale Tumoren im Erwachsenenalter. Teil 2: Extraaxiale Tumoren. Radiologe 2002; 42: 840–855

Kleihues P et al. WHO Classification of Tumours. Pathology and Genetics. Tumours of the nervous system. International Agency for Research of Cancer. Library Cataloguing in Publication Data. 2000: 129–137

Tumors

Definition

▶ **Etiology, pathophysiology, pathogenesis**
Disseminated clumps of cells • Malformation of organ differentiation.
Dermoid: Keratinous inclusion mass • Contains epidermal tissue along with fat, hair, calcification, and sweat glands.
Teratoma: Cells from all three germ layers • Localization: pineal region, suprasellar region.
Hamartoma: Congenital, nonneoplastic ectopic tissue • Neuronal tissue. Localization: temporal lobe, suprasellar region.
Lipoma: Contains fat.

Imaging Signs

▶ **Modality of choice**
MRI.
▶ **CT**
Density of the tumors depend on their histologic composition.
Lipoma: Hypodense to brain tissue with density around – 100 HU.
Dermoid: Hypodense to brain tissue with density around – 100 HU • May include calcifications.
Hamartoma: Can escape detection on CT • Larger findings are slightly hypodense to surrounding brain tissue.
Teratoma: Density varies with the specific composition • Components are isodense to fat and occasionally calcifications are present.
▶ **MRI**
Does not enhance.
Lipoma: Homogeneously hyperintense on T2-weighted and T1-weighted images.
Dermoid: Inhomogeneous signal with hyperintense (fatty) and hypointense areas (calcification) • Dermoid components isointense to fat may be detected in the subarachnoid space secondary to rupture.
Hamartoma: Isointense to brain tissue • No perifocal edema • T1-weighted image inversion recovery sequence is useful.
Teratoma: Inhomogeneous signal intensity, depending on the specific histologic composition.

Clinical Aspects

▶ **Typical presentation**
Unspecific symptoms • Seizure • Obstructed CSF flow • Tumors of the pituitary stalk can lead to precocious puberty.
▶ **Treatment options**
Surgical removal • Where there is involvement of the pineal body, obstructed CSF flow is treated symptomatically with a shunt or ventriculostomy.

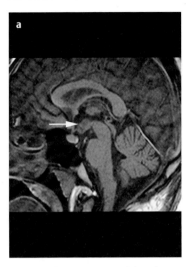
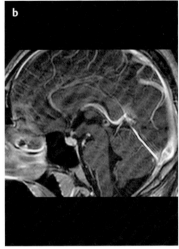

Fig. 6.35 a, b Hamartoma of the tuber cinereum (arrow). Sagittal T1-weighted MR images before (**a**) and after (**b**) contrast administration. Nonenhancing lesion with mass effect, isointense to gray matter.

▶ **Course and prognosis**
As these are benign tumors, prognosis depends on the symptoms (seizure or obstructed CSF flow).

▶ **What does the clinician want to know?**
Localization ● Extent ● Diagnosis of type.

Differential Diagnosis

Pineal tumors	– Germinomas and pineoblastomas enhance
Sella	– Craniopharyngioma: can enhance
	– Rathke cleft cyst: cystic component, never contains fat
Arachnoid cyst	– Always isointense and isodense to fluid
	– Never contains fat
Colloid cyst	– Usually only slightly hyperintense on T1-weighted MR images (dermoid and lipoma are strongly hyperintense)

Tips and Pitfalls

Misinterpreting a tumor of the tuber cinereum as a normal mammillary body.

Fig. 6.36 Ruptured dermoid cyst. Axial T1-weighted MR image. Structures isointense to fat in the subarachnoid space, remnants of the fatty contents of a dermoid cyst.

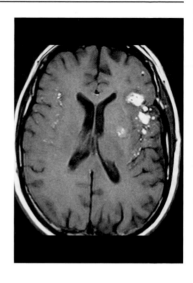

Selected References

Grunwald I et al. Intrazerebrale Tumoren im Erwachsenenalter. Teil 2: Extraaxiale Tumoren. Radiologe 2002; 42: 840–855

Mader I et al. Die kernspintomographische Differentialdiagnose von Tumoren der Pinealisregion. Klinische Neuroradiologie 2001; 11 (1): 25–32

Definition

▶ **Epidemiology**
Prevalence: 0.24% ● *Sex predilection:* Males ● *Peak age:* 0–20 and 30–50 years.
▶ **Etiology, pathophysiology, pathogenesis**
Well demarcated intra-axial tumor of the ventricular ependyma ● Supratentorial
(30% of all cases) or infratentorial (70%) ● Histologic findings include perivascu-
lar pseudo-rosettes and ependymal rosettes ● Mitoses are minimal or absent ●
Necrosis can also occur in WHO grade II tumors.

Imaging Signs

▶ **Modality of choice**
MRI.
▶ **CT findings**
Inhomogeneous tumor ● Close proximity to ventricular system ● Clarifications
are rare ● No perifocal edema.
▶ **MRI findings**
Close proximity to ventricular system ● Hyperintense to surrounding brain tis-
sue on T2-weighted and FLAIR images ● No perifocal edema, although there may
be significant compression of the ventricular system with obstructed CSF flow ●
Non-contrast-enhanced T1-weighted images show a hypointense tumor whose
signal intensity increases significantly and inhomogeneously after contrast administration ● Drop metastases can occur throughout the entire cerebrospinal
CSF space; therefore, MRI examination of the entire central nervous system is indicated.

Clinical Aspects

▶ **Typical presentation**
Unspecific ● Obstructed CSF flow: headache, nausea, and vomiting ● Neurologic
deficits are rare.
▶ **Treatment options**
Surgical removal ● Radiation therapy ● Shunt where flow of CSF is obstructed.
▶ **Course and prognosis**
Prognosis varies with WHO grade ● Healing is possible in the absence of drop
metastases.
▶ **What does the clinician want to know?**
Localization ● Extent ● Drop metastases along the axis of the central nervous
system ● Differential diagnosis.

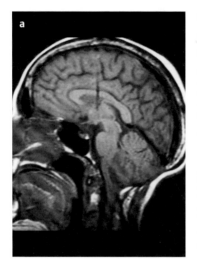 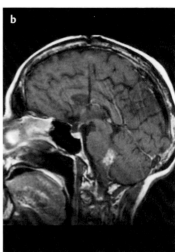

Fig. 6.37a, b Ependymoma of the fourth ventricle. Sagittal T1-weighted MR image before (**a**) and after (**b**) contrast administration. The superior portions of the inhomogeneous tumor on the non-contrast-enhanced image enhance significantly after administration of contrast. The obstructed CSF flow that invariably occurs with a tumor in this location is treated by CSF diverting procedure.

Differential Diagnosis

Medulloblastoma	– Arises in cerebellum
	– Differential diagnosis can be difficult because even medulloblastomas vary in their enhancement and form drop metastases via the CSF
Glioblastoma	– Usually marked perifocal edema
	– Acute symptoms, usually with seizure
	– Elevated rrCBV, 2–3 times normal
Pilocytic astrocytoma	– Usually unilateral asymmetrical ring enhancement
	– Not adjacent to ventricular system
Epidermoid	– Hypointense on T1-weighted MR images
	– Does not enhance
	– Pronounced diffusion restriction

Tips and Pitfalls

Failing to examine brain and spinal cord completely and missing metastases as a result.

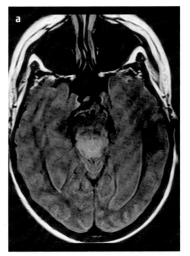

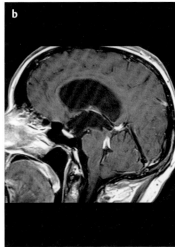

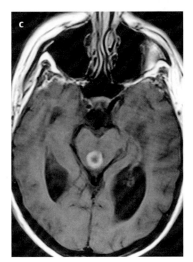

Fig. 6.38 a–c Ependymoma of the aqueduct of Sylvius. Axial proton-density image (**a**), sagittal (**b**) and axial (**c**) T1-weighted MR images after contrast administration. Significant enhancement is seen especially of the tumor components in the vicinity of the CSF space. The hyperintensity in the pons suggests brainstem involvement.

Selected References

Reith W et al. Supratentorielle Tumoren im Kindesalter. Radiologe 2003; 43: 986–996
Grunwald I et al. Intrazerebrale Tumoren im Erwachsenenalter. Teil 1: Intraaxiale Tumoren. Radiologe 2002; 42: 571–587

Definition (Ganglioglioma, Dysembryoplastic Neuroepithelial Tumor [DNT])

▶ **Epidemiology**
Incidence: 1.3 % of all brain tumors ● *Sex predilection:* M:F = 1:2 ● *Peak age:* 0–30 years.

▶ **Etiology, pathophysiology, pathogenesis**
The tumor can occur in all sections of the brain at cortical and subcortical locations ● The temporal lobe is affected particularly often.
Histology:
Ganglioglioma: Irregular arrangement of multipolar, dysplastic neurons ● No necrosis ● Low rate of mitosis.
DNT: Column-like arrangements of oligodendrocytes surrounded by an eosinophilic matrix ● Low rate of mitosis ● Malignant degeneration is very rare.

Imaging Signs

▶ **Modality of choice**
MRI.

▶ **CT findings**
Ganglioglioma: Isodense to hyperdense solid tumor ● Can exhibit a component isodense to fluid ● Calcifications are rare.
DNT: Hypodense tumor ● Calcifications occur in up to 30 % of all lesions ● Cortical location.

▶ **MRI findings**
Ganglioglioma: Hyperintense on T2-weighted and FLAIR images and hypointense on the T1-weighted image ● Variable enhancement ● Slight or absent perifocal edema ● Imaging findings can contribute decisively to a differential diagnosis of lesions in typical locations.
DNT: Hyperintense on T2-weighted and FLAIR images and hypointense on the T1-weighted image ● Does not enhance.

Clinical Aspects

▶ **Typical presentation**
Seizure.

▶ **Treatment options**
Surgical resection ● Anticonvulsant therapy.

▶ **Course and prognosis**
Medical management of seizures is often sufficient ● Complete healing is possible with total resection ● Malignant degeneration is rare.

▶ **What does the clinician want to know?**
Localization ● Extent ● Differential diagnosis (important because histologic findings in ganglioglioma are not always unequivocal).

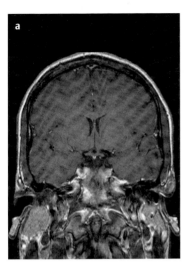 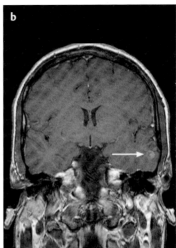

Fig. 6.39 a, b Ganglioglioma of the left temporal lobe. Coronal T1-weighted MR images before (**a**) and after (**b**) contrast administration. The tumor lies in the cortex, and its caudal portion enhances (arrow).

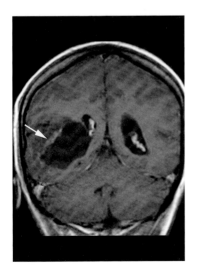

Fig. 6.40 Ganglioglioma of the right temporal lobe. Coronal T1-weighted MR image after contrast administration. Aside from an enhancing solid component (arrow), there is a large tumor cyst which compresses the right lateral ventricle.

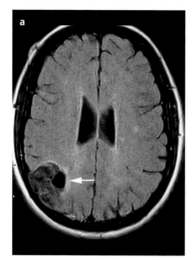

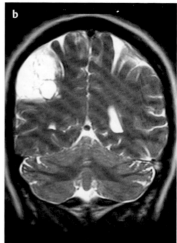

Fig. 6.41 a–c DNT of the right parietal lobe. Axial FLAIR image (**a**), T1-weighted MR image after contrast administration (**c**), and coronal T2-weighted MR image (**b**). The tumor consists of a solid component and a cystic component (arrow). The cortical location and lack of enhancement are typical. The tumor has led to thinning of the skull (**b**).

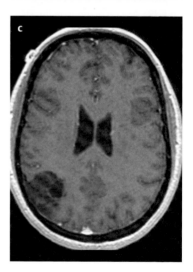

Differential Diagnosis

Hamartoma	– Isointense to brain tissue
Pilocytic astrocytoma	– Differential diagnosis can be difficult
	– Usually not located in cortex

Tips and Pitfalls

Evaluating enhancement as a sign of malignancy.

Selected References

Reith W et al. Supratentorielle Tumoren im Kindesalter. Radiologe 2003; 43: 986–996

Kleihues P et al. WHO Classification of Tumours. Pathology and Genetics. Tumours of the nervous system. International Agency for Research of Cancer. Library Cataloguing in Publication Data. 2000: 129–137

Tumors

Definition

▶ **Epidemiology**
Incidence in the population: 0.11 % ● No sex predilection ● *Peak age:* 20–30 years.

▶ **Etiology, pathophysiology, pathogenesis**
WHO grade I tumor ● Consists of stromal cells and capillaries ● Twenty-five percent of all cases occur in association with von Hippel–Lindau disease (hamartomas, renal carcinoma) ● Tumors are usually infratentorial, especially those associated with von Hippel–Lindau disease.

Imaging Signs

▶ **Modality of choice**
MRI and angiography.

▶ **CT findings**
Tumor isodense to CSF ● Solid component of variable size (asymmetrical, marginal position) ● Complications: hemorrhaging, obstructed CSF flow.

▶ **MRI findings**
Tumor appears hyperdense on T2-weighted images and hypointense on T1-weighted images ● Contrast images show eccentric, significantly enhancing tumor component ● As hemangioblastomas can occur as multilocular lesions, examination of the brain and spinal cord is indicated in all cases.

▶ **Angiography findings**
Significant contrast enhancement ● Early venous filling.

Clinical Aspects

▶ **Typical presentation**
Usually asymptomatic because tumor is slow-growing ● Obstructed CSF flow ● Secondary polycythemia resulting from erythropoietin production.

▶ **Treatment options**
Surgical resection.

▶ **Course and prognosis**
Prognosis is good ● In von Hippel–Lindau disease (see p. 270), hemangioblastoma is the second most common cause of death after renal cell carcinoma ● However, mean survival time is minimally reduced.

▶ **What does the clinician want to know?**
Site ● Extent ● Obstructed CSF flow ● Diagnosis of type ● Spinal involvement.

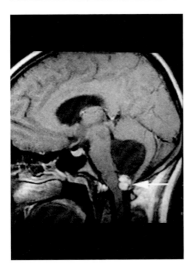

Fig. 6.42 Hemangioblastoma of the cerebellar vermis. Sagittal T1-weighted MR image after IV contrast administration. Large cystic hypointense tumor component that fills the fourth ventricle and smaller enhancing tumor component (arrow).

Differential Diagnosis

Pilocytic astrocytoma	– Children or adolescents – Unilocular; hemangioblastomas are often multilocular
Glioblastoma	– rrCBV elevated to twice normal – Usually ring enhancement – Pronounced perifocal edema – Age over 45 years
Abscess	– Clinical findings – Usually pronounced diffusion restriction – Pronounced perifocal edema
Metastasis	– History – Perifocal edema – Restricted diffusion may be present

Tips and Pitfalls

Failing to examine brain and spinal cord completely.

Fig. 6.43 Coronal DSA after injection of the left vertebral artery. Heavily vascularized caudal tumor component showing significant tumor blush.

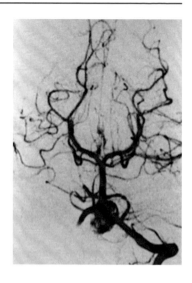

Selected References

Choyke P et al. Von Hippel-Lindau disease: genetic, clinical and imaging features. Radiology 1995; 194 (3): 629–642

Sora S et al. Incidence of von Hippel-Lindau Disease in Hemangioblastoma Patients: The University of Tokyo Hospital Experience from 1954–1998. Acta Neurochirurgica 2000; 143 (9): 893–896

Definition

▶ **Epidemiology**
No sex predilection ● *Peak age:* 40–60 years.
▶ **Etiology, pathophysiology, pathogenesis**
Diffuse gliomatous tumor ● Involvement of at least two cerebral lobes ● Histology: Astrocytes with oval or fusiform, usually hyperchromatic nuclei ● No microvascular proliferation.

Imaging Signs

▶ **Modality of choice**
MRI.
▶ **CT findings**
Tumor with a homogeneous internal structure ● Mass effect (subfalcial herniation, narrowing of the cisterns, reduced delineation of the cerebral cortex) ● Hemorrhages are rare ● Usually no calcifications.
▶ **MRI findings**
Homogeneously increased signal on T2-weighted and FLAIR images ● Slightly hypointense to normal brain tissue on T1-weighted images ● Bilateral or infratentorial involvement is possible ● No contrast enhancement ● Usually increases rapidly in size within a few months.

Clinical Aspects

▶ **Typical presentation**
Clinical symptoms are usually unspecific ● Pyramidal tract signs ● Progressive dementia ● Headache.
▶ **Treatment options**
Limited ● Radiation therapy may be attempted.
▶ **Course and prognosis**
Approximately 50% of patients die within 12 months.
▶ **What does the clinician want to know?**
Diagnosis of type ● Extent ● Localization ● Differential diagnosis from gliomas.

Fig. 6.44 Gliomatosis cerebri. Axial T2-weighted MR image. Involvement of the frontal and temporal lobes. Diffuse, homogeneous hyperintensity especially in the medulla.

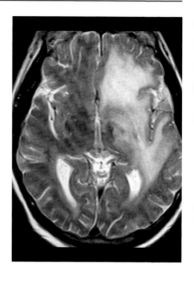

Differential Diagnosis

Low-grade astrocytoma	– Difficult to differentiate, especially in beginning gliomatosis
Low-grade oligodendrogliomas	– Increased rrCBV – Calcifications can occur
Higher grade gliomas	– Abnormal enhancement – Greatly increased rrCBV
Leukodystrophies	– Usually bilateral in the vicinity of the ventricular system – No mass effect
Encephalitis	– Abnormal CSF findings – Usually abnormal enhancement

Tips and Pitfalls

Misinterpreting as a low-grade astrocytoma.

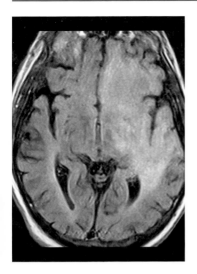

Fig. 6.45 Axial FLAIR image. Involvement of the frontal and temporal lobes (same case as Fig. 6.**44**).

Selected References

Hartmann M et al. Funktionelle MR-Verfahren in der Diagnostik intraaxialer Hirntumoren: Perfusions- und Diffusionbildgebung. Rofo Fortschr Geb Rontgenstr Neuen Bildgeb Verfahr 2002; 174: 955–964

Jennings MT et al. Gliomatosis cerebri presenting as intractable epilepsy during early childhood. J Child Neurol 1995; 10: 37–45

Definition

▶ **Epidemiology**
Incidence: 0.5% of all intracranial tumors ● No sex predilection ● No peak age.
▶ **Etiology, pathophysiology, pathogenesis**
Benign tumor ● Arises from the choroid plexus of the ventricular system ● Choroid plexus papillomas (WHO grade I) are distinguished from choroid plexus carcinomas (WHO grades III and IV) ● In children and adolescents they occur primarily in the lateral ventricles; in adults primarily in the third and fourth ventricles.

Imaging Signs

▶ **Modality of choice**
MRI.
▶ **CT findings**
Moderately hyperdense tumor ● Widening of the ventricular system ● Tumors in the fourth ventricle or interventricular foramen of Monro lead to obstructed CSF flow ● Tumor spread is limited to the ventricular system.
▶ **MRI findings**
Tumor is hypointense or isointense to brain tissue on T1-weighted images, hyperintense on T2-weighted images ● Enhances significantly ● Well demarcated.

Clinical Aspects

▶ **Typical presentation**
Signs of obstructed CSF flow: Headache ● Nausea ● Vomiting ● Vertigo ● Papilledema ● Rarely the tumor causes hypersecretion of CSF.
▶ **Treatment options**
Surgical resection ● A CSF shunt is indicated only in inoperable tumors.
▶ **Course and prognosis**
Prognosis for total resection is good.
▶ **What does the clinician want to know?**
Localization ● Extent ● Does the tumor cross the borders of the ventricular system? ● Obstructed CSF flow.

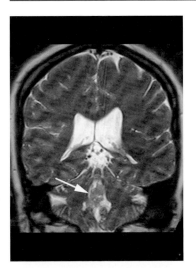

Fig. 6.46 Choroid plexus papilloma. Coronal T2-weighted MR image. Hypointense tumor in the fourth ventricle (arrow).

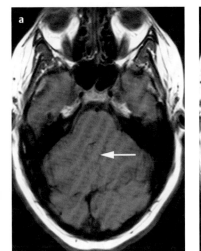 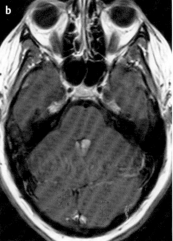

Fig. 6.47a, b Axial T1-weighted MR image before (**a**) and after (**b**) contrast administration. The tumor is isointense to brain tissue on the non-contrast-enhanced image (**a**, arrow) and enhances significantly (**b**). Unlike a choroid plexus carcinoma, it does not cross the borders of the ventricular system. Same case as Fig. 6.**46**.

Differential Diagnosis

Choroid plexus carcinoma	– Differential diagnosis can be difficult
	– Crosses the borders of the ventricular system
	– Perifocal edema
	– Inhomogeneous enhancement
	– Signal behavior identical to WHO grade I tumors
Subependymoma	– Usually enhances minimally or not at all
Intraventricular meningioma	– Differential diagnosis can be difficult or impossible
	– Usually isointense to brain tissue on T2-weighted MR images

Tips and Pitfalls

Misinterpreting the lesions as choroid plexus cysts.

Selected References

Grunwald I et al. Intrazerebrale Tumoren im Erwachsenenalter. Teil 2: Extraaxiale Tumoren. Radiologe 2002; 42: 840–855

Taylor MB et al. Magnetic resonance imaging in the diagnosis and management of choroid plexus carcinoma in children. Pediatric Radiology 2001; 31: 624–630

Definition

▶ **Epidemiology**
  Incidence: Approximately 0.5 % ● In 50 % of all cases, in the vicinity of the sylvian fissure.
▶ **Etiology, pathophysiology, pathogenesis**
  Local widening of the subarachnoid space ● Developmental anomaly of the arachnoid (duplication) ● Closed and communicating cysts can occur.

Imaging Signs

▶ **Modality of choice**
  MRI.
▶ **Findings on plain skull radiography**
  In most cases there are no abnormal findings ● Large arachnoid cysts may produce compressive thinning of the skull, skull deformation, and/or signs of chronically increased intracranial pressure.
▶ **CT findings**
  Often an incidental finding ● Homogeneous hypodense cyst contents ● No enhancement ● Regional compressive thinning of the skull ● Significant displacement of adjacent brain structures may occur without any symptoms.
▶ **Cisternography findings**
  Verifies whether the cyst communicates with the CSF space.
  Examination procedure: A plain CT of the skull is obtained before intrathecal injection of contrast agent ● A second CT of the skull is obtained immediately after injection, as are further studies with measurement of the ROI 2, 6, and 24 hours later ● Density increases over time where the cyst communicates with the CSF space.
▶ **MRI findings**
  A frequent incidental finding ● Typical signal isointense to CSF: hypointense to brain tissue on FLAIR image, hypointense on T1-weighted image, hyperintense on T2-weighted image, hypointense on diffusion-weighted image ● No enhancement on the T1-weighted image after contrast administration ● Cine MR may be used to measure CSF flow to evaluate communication between cyst and subarachnoid space (caution: low flow rate; select correct direction of phase coding) ● Temporopolar false-positive findings may occur due to the proximity of the internal carotid artery ● When the MRI criteria are fulfilled, findings are diagnostic of an arachnoid cyst.

Clinical Aspects

▶ **Typical presentation**
  Usually asymptomatic ● Rarely symptoms of increased intracranial pressure may occur (headache, nausea, vomiting, vertigo, papilledema with impaired vision, rarely epileptogenic focus).

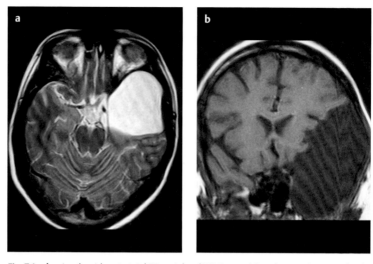

Fig. 7.1 a, b Arachnoid cyst. Axial T2-weighted MR image (**a**) and coronal T1-weighted MR image (**b**). Temporopolar arachnoid cyst with a signal isointense to CSF.

▶ **Treatment options**
Invasive diagnostic studies are not usually indicated as the majority of arachnoid cysts are not clinically significant • Complicated cysts that affect CSF flow may be treated with a shunt.

▶ **Course and prognosis**
Prognosis is usually favorable.

▶ **What does the clinician want to know?**
Diagnosis of type • Differential diagnosis excluding epidermoid and large cerebromedullary cistern • Communication with CSF space • Change in size on follow-up studies.

Differential Diagnosis

Epidermoid	– Hyperintense on the FLAIR and diffusion-weighted MR images
Cholesteatoma	– Isointense on the T1-weighted MR image
Cystic meningioma	– Ring enhancement

Tips and Pitfalls

Misinterpreting the lesion as an epidermoid.

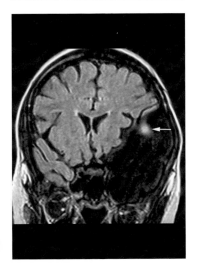

Fig. 7.2 Coronal FLAIR image. Deformation and thinning of the skull due to compression from the arachnoid cyst. Slight CSF flow artifact along the superior margin of the cyst (arrow).

Selected References

Sommer I et al. Congenital supratentoriell arachnoidal and giant cysts in children: a clinical study with arguments for a conservative approach. Child's nervous system 1997; 13 (1): 8–12

Ibarra R et al. Role of MRI in the diagnosis of complicated arachnoid cyst. Pediatric Radiology 2000; 30 (5): 329–331

Gizewski E et.al.: Epidermoid oder Arachnoidalzyste: CISS, FLAIR und Diffusionsbilder als Ausweg aus dem diagnostischen Dilemma. Rofo Fortschr Geb Rontgenstr Neuen Bildgeb Verfahr 2001; 173: 77–78

Cysts

Definition

▶ **Epidemiology**
Localization: Anterior perforated substance (posterior to the amygdala) ● Mesencephalon (crus cerebri) ● White matter of the cerebral hemispheres (centrum semiovale).
Peak age: Basal location in young patients ● At the convexity with increasing age (sign of decreasing brain volume).

▶ **Etiology, pathophysiology, pathogenesis**
Extensions of the subarachnoid space filled with CSF surround the arterioles and veins passing through the cortex and white matter down to the capillary level.

Imaging Signs

▶ **Modality of choice**
CT or MRI.

▶ **CT findings**
Typical localization (basal region, mesencephalon, convexity) ● Isodense to CSF ● Size ranges from a few millimeters to several centimeters ● No enhancement ● No mass effect or shrinkage ● Large lesions may exhibit septate structure.

▶ **MRI findings**
Typical localization (see above) ● Hypointense to brain tissue on T1-weighted and FLAIR images ● Hyperintense to brain tissue on T2-weighted images ● No enhancement.

Clinical Aspects

▶ **Typical presentation**
Usually an incidental finding ● Virchow–Robin cysts with mass effect are rare but may obstruct the flow of CSF where they do occur ● In such cases, patients typically present with symptoms of increased intracranial pressure: headache, nausea, vomiting, vertigo, papilledema.

▶ **Treatment options**
Lesions are further clinically significant only where complications are present.

▶ **Course and prognosis**
Favorable.

▶ **What does the clinician want to know?**
Differentiate from other abnormal findings ● "Leave me alone" lesion.

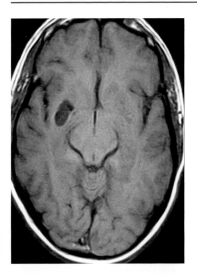

Fig. 7.3 Expanded Virchow–Robin space. Axial T1-weighted MR image. Hypointensity in the right putamen.

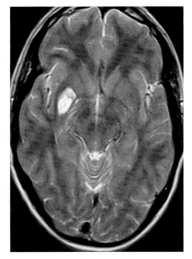

Fig. 7.4 Axial T2-weighted MR image. Virchow–Robin space hyperintense to brain tissue (patient from Fig. 7.**3**).

Cysts

Differential Diagnosis

Lacunae	– Different localization: basal ganglia, internal capsule, medulla
Inflammation	– FLAIR images: hyperintense
Parasites	– Different localization
	– May enhance
	– Calcification may occur
Neurosarcoidosis	– Enhances
Arachnoid cysts	– Lie outside the brain tissue
Epidermoid	– FLAIR and diffusion-weighted MR images: hyperintense

Tips and Pitfalls

Misinterpreting as a lacunar infarction.

Selected References

Adachi M et al. Dilated Virchow–Robin spaces. MRI pathological study. Neuroradiology 1998; 40: 27–31

Bokura H et al. Distinguishing silent lacunar infarction from enlarged Virchow Robin spaces: a MRI and pathological study. Journal of Neurology 1998; 245 (2): 116–122

Papayannis C et al. Expanding Virchow Robin Spaces in the midbrain causing hydrocephalus. AJNR 2003; 24: 1399–1403

Definition

▶ **Epidemiology**
Incidence: Approximately 2% ● *Sex predilection:* Females ● *Peak age:* 20–30 years.
▶ **Etiology, pathophysiology, pathogenesis**
Histology: Glial pineal cyst ● Usually an incidental finding.

Imaging Signs

▶ **Modality of choice**
MRI.
▶ **CT findings**
Enlargement of the pineal gland ● Hypodense homogeneous internal structure.
▶ **MRI findings**
Enlargement of the pineal gland ● T1-weighted image: isointense to brain tissue at the margin, hypointense in the center ● T2-weighted image: hyperintense to brain tissue ● FLAIR image: hyperintense to brain tissue ● Capsular pattern of enhancement.

Clinical Aspects

▶ **Typical presentation**
Usually asymptomatic ● Rarely signs of obstructed CSF flow: headache, nausea, vomiting, vertigo, oculomotor disturbance ● Parinaud syndrome: vertical gaze palsy.
▶ **Therapeutic options**
Obstructed CSF flow is treated with shunt or ventriculostomy.
▶ **Course and prognosis**
Favorable ● Usually requires no treatment.
▶ **What does the clinician want to know?**
Diagnosis of type ● Obstructed CSF flow?

Differential Diagnosis

Pineocytoma	– Difficult differential diagnosis where only a portion of the original pineal tissue is identifiable
	– Enhances significantly
	– Calcifications may be visualized on CT
Other pineal tumors	– Enhancement
	– Solid tumor component
	– Obstructed CSF flow

Fig. 7.5 Pineal cyst. Coronal T1-weighted MR image after contrast administration. Round cyst in the pineal region with slight linear enhancement of the cyst wall and/or displaced pineal tissue (arrow).

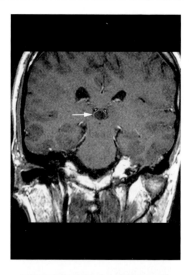

Fig. 7.6 Coronal FLAIR image. Signal is hyperintense to CSF (arrow) because the protein content is higher than that of CSF. Same case as Fig. 7.**5**.

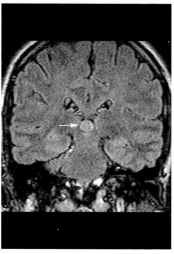

Tips and Pitfalls

Misinterpreting as a solid pineal tumor • No follow-up, because there are also purely cystic pineal tumors.

Selected References

Mader I et al. Die kernspintomographische Differentialdiagnose von Tumoren der Pinealisregion. Klinische Neuroradiologie 2001; 11 (1): 25–32

Michielsen G et al. Symptomatic pineal cysts: clinical manifestations and management. Acta Neurochir (Vienna) 2002; 144 (3): 233–242

Definition

▶ **Epidemiology**
Frequency: 3.2 per million • *Occurrence:* 0.2–2% of all intracranial tumors • *Peak age:* Usually in adults.

▶ **Etiology, pathophysiology, pathogenesis**
Cyst usually located in the ventricular system • Benign tumor • Primary localization: third ventricle • Histology: small columns of ciliated epithelium arising from the basal membrane and covered by the glycocalyx • The cyst wall secretes a turbid yellowish fluid into the cyst.

Imaging Signs

▶ **Modality of choice**
MRI.

▶ **CT findings**
Density and size can vary within short intervals • Smoothly demarcated • Homogeneous • Usually hyperdense • Dilatation of the third ventricle. The interventricular foramina of Monro are displaced laterally • Blockage of the interventricular foramen of Monro leads to obstructed CSF flow with widening of the lateral ventricles.

▶ **MRI findings**
Lesion may exhibit variable signal intensity • Typically hyperintense to brain tissue on T1-weighted images • Signal intensity varies relative to brain tissue on T2-weighted images • Hyperintense to brain tissue on FLAIR and proton density images • Only slight ring enhancement • Obstructed CSF flow.

Clinical Aspects

▶ **Typical presentation**
Headache • Nausea • Vomiting • Vertigo • Papilledema.

▶ **Treatment options**
Surgical removal • Shunt.

▶ **Course and prognosis**
Prognosis for surgical removal is good • The size and composition of the cyst contents can change rapidly (obstructed CSF flow, impingement due to acute blockage of the foramen of Monro).

▶ **What does the clinician want to know?**
Diagnosis of type • Localization • Extent • Change in size • Obstructed CSF flow.

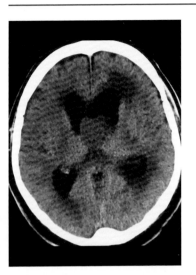

Fig. 7.7 Colloid cyst. Axial CT. Cyst in the roof of the third ventricle at the interventricular foramen of Monro, hyperdense to CSF.

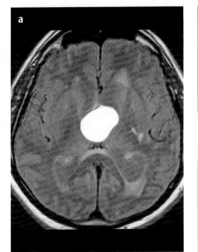

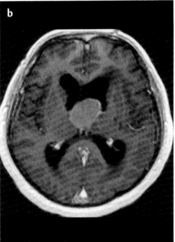

Fig. 7.8 a, b Axial proton density image (**a**) and T1-weighted MR image (**b**) after contrast administration. The higher protein content of the cysts produces the hyperintense internal signal. Ring enhancement after contrast administration. Same case as Fig. 7.**7**.

Differential Diagnosis

Arachnoid cyst	– Signal and density identical to CSF
	– Does not enhance
Cyst of the septum pellucidum	– Central
	– Long
	– Signal and density identical to CSF
	– Does not enhance

Tips and Pitfalls

Misinterpreting as an arachnoid cyst.

Selected References

Armao CM et al. Colloid cyst of the 3 rd ventricle: Imaging-pathologic correlation. AJNR 2000; 21: 1470–1477

Büttner A et al. Colloid cyst of the 3 rd ventricle with fatal outcome: a report of two cases and review of the literature. Int J Legal Med 1997; 110: 260–266

Kachara R et al. Changing characteristics of a colloid cyst of the 3 rd ventrikel. Neuroradiology 1999; 41: 188–189

Veerman E et al. On the chemical characterization of colloid cyst contents. Acta Neurochir (Vienna) 1998; 140: 303–307

Definition

▶ **Epidemiology**
Incidence at autopsy: 13–22% ● Symptomatic Rathke cleft cysts are rare ● Up to 1991, 147 cases were described in the literature ● *Sex predilection:* M:F = 1:2 ● *Peak age:* 50–60 years.
▶ **Etiology, pathophysiology, pathogenesis**
Vestige of the Rathke cleft, arising from a part of the embryonic craniopharyngeal duct ● Usually in the suprasellar region, less often in the infrasellar region ● Histology is variable: cubic or cylindrical, mucilaginous or ciliated.

Imaging Signs

▶ **Modality of choice**
MRI.
▶ **CT findings**
Round cyst ● Hypodense or isodense ● Does not enhance.
▶ **MRI findings**
Smoothly demarcated ● Hypointense to isointense to brain tissue on T1-weighted images, depending on protein content, and hyperintense on T2-weighted images ● Cyst wall enhances slightly.

Clinical Aspects

▶ **Typical presentation**
Usually asymptomatic ● Symptomatic Rathke cleft cysts exhibit clinical symptoms similar to pituitary adenomas ● Impaired vision ● Obstructed CSF flow ● Headache ● Galactorrhea ● Amenorrhea ● Hypopituitarism.
▶ **Treatment options**
Surgical resection.
▶ **Course and prognosis**
Usually an incidental finding ● Few lesions recur after surgery.
▶ **What does the clinician want to know?**
Differential diagnosis excluding craniopharyngioma, arachnoid cyst, and pituitary adenoma ● Compression of optic chiasm ● Progression.

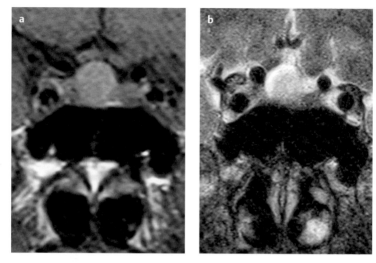

Fig. 7.9 a, b Rathke cleft cyst. Coronal T1-weighted MR image (**a**) and T2-weighted MR image (**b**). Lesion hyperintense to the adenohypophysis extending into the intrasellar and suprasellar regions and displacing the optic chiasm. The adenohypophysis is compressed to the left and right of it but otherwise normal. The left part of the cyst is hypo-intense to the rest of the pituitary tissue on the T2-weighted image (**b**).

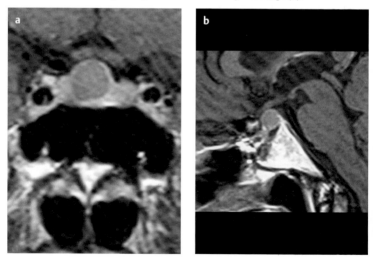

Fig. 7.10 a, b Coronal (**a**) and sagittal (**b**) T1-weighted MR images after contrast administration. Cyst wall enhances, cyst contents do not (patient from Fig. 7.**9**).

Differential Diagnosis

Craniopharyngioma	– Differential diagnosis can be difficult especially with small craniopharyngiomas
	– Calcifications on CT suggest craniopharyngioma
	– Solid component enhances significantly
	– Recurrence
Pituitary adenoma	– Intrasellar origin
	– Large adenomas have inhomogeneous internal structure
Granulomatous disorders	– Significant, homogeneous enhancement
Metastases	– Significant enhancement

Tips and Pitfalls

Misinterpreting as pituitary adenoma • Failing to consider Rathke cleft cyst.

Selected References

Saeki N et al. MRI findings and clinical manifestations in Rathke's Cleft Cyst. Acta Neurochir (Vienna) 1999; 141: 1055–1061

Definition

▶ **Epidemiology**
Often detectable even in children ● Usually an incidental finding.

▶ **Etiology, pathophysiology, pathogenesis**
Arises from embryonic neuroepithelium ● Cyst contents: CSF with varying protein content.

Imaging Signs

▶ **Modality of choice**
MRI.

▶ **CT findings**
Asymmetrical enlargement of one ventricle ● Hypodense enlarged choroid plexus ● Cyst does not enhance.

▶ **MRI findings**
Usually an incidental finding ● T1-weighted image: hypointense to brain tissue ● T2-weighted and FLAIR images: hyperintense to brain tissue, may even be brighter than CSF depending on protein content ● Diffusion-weighted image: strongly hyperintense to brain tissue ● No enhancement in the cyst itself but marginal enhancement in the choroid plexus.

Clinical Aspects

▶ **Typical presentation**
Usually an incidental finding ● CSF flow is only rarely obstructed.

▶ **Treatment options**
Only required for obstructed CSF flow ● Shunt or ventriculostomy.

▶ **Course and prognosis**
Usually requires no treatment.

▶ **What does the clinician want to know?**
Exclude choroid plexus papilloma and carcinoma ● Obstructed CSF flow.

Differential Diagnosis

Choroid plexus papilloma	– Enhancement in the center of the lesion and on DSA
Choroid plexus carcinoma	– Significant enhancement in the center of the lesion as well
	– Infiltration of the adjacent parts of the brain as well
	– Flow of CSF is usually obstructed
	– Often occurs in children

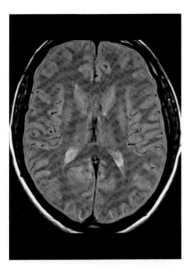

Fig. 7.11 Choroid plexus cyst. Axial proton density image. Smoothly demarcated cyst hyperintense to brain tissue in the posterior horn of the right lateral ventricle. CSF flow is unobstructed and there is no perifocal edema.

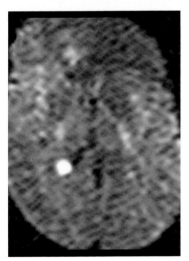

Fig. 7.12 Axial diffusion-weighted MR image. Significant restriction to diffusion in the choroid plexus cyst (right).

Tips and Pitfalls

Misinterpreting as a choroid plexus tumor.

Selected References

Parizek J. et al. Choroid plexus cyst of the left lateral ventricle with intermittent blockage of the foramen of Monro, and intitial invagination into the III. ventricle in a child. Child's Nerv Syst 1998; 14: 700–708

Radaideh M. et al. Unusual small choroid plexus cyst obstructing the Foramen of Monroe: Case report. AJNR 2002; 23: 841–843

Definition
▶ **Etiology, pathophysiology, pathogenesis**
Diffuse carcinomatous infiltration of the meninges and ependyma in the presence of a known primary tumor.

Imaging Signs
▶ **Modality of choice**
MRI.
▶ **CT findings**
Plain CT usually detects only secondary signs (obstructed CSF flow) • Increased meningeal enhancement is seen after IV contrast administration.
▶ **MRI findings**
T1-weighted and T2-weighted images usually show only secondary signs (cerebral edema, obstructed CSF flow) • FLAIR images how increased signal intensity of the subarachnoid space consistent with meningeal involvement and increased protein content in CSF • On T1-weighted images after contrast administration, the meninges show a diffuse increase in signal intensity • The meningeal cover layer of cranial nerves enhances • Ependymal enhancement.

Clinical Aspects
▶ **Typical presentation**
Late symptom of a tumor disorder • Patients are severely ill • Signs of obstructed CSF flow.
▶ **Treatment options**
Intrathecal chemotherapy • Radiation therapy.
▶ **Course and prognosis**
Extremely poor • Depends on the type of primary tumor • Survival time is usually only a few weeks.
▶ **What does the clinician want to know?**
Confirmation of tentative diagnosis • Obstructed CSF flow.

Differential Diagnosis

Meningitis	– Differential diagnosis is not possible on the basis of imaging findings – CSF, clinical symptoms – History
Granulomatous disorders	– Nodular enhancement – CSF findings – Differential diagnosis on the basis of imaging findings can be difficult
Acute subarachnoid hemorrhage	– Does not enhance

Fig. 8.1 Meningeal carcinomatosis. Axial T1-weighted MR image after contrast administration. Enhancement in the leptomeninges on the surface of the cerebellum (arrow).

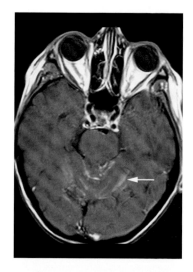

Fig. 8.2 Coronal T1-weighted MR image after contrast administration. Infratentorial pial and dural enhancement (lower arrow). Subependymal enhancement in the posterior horn of the left lateral ventricle (upper arrow).

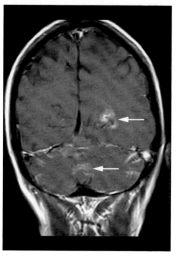

Tips and Pitfalls

Obtaining only axial T1-weighted MR images after contrast administration ● Meningeal enhancement is better visualized on coronal and sagittal views.

Selected References

Grunwald I et al. Intrazerebrale Tumoren im Erwachsenenalter. Teil 2: Extraaxiale Tumoren. Radiologe 2002; 42: 840–855

Tsuchiya K et al. FLAIR MRI for Diagnosing Intracranial Meningeal Carcinomatosis. AJR 2001; 176: 1585–1588

Definition

▶ **Etiology, pathophysiology, pathogenesis**
Reactive irritation of the meninges following surgery or lumbar puncture • No signs of inflammation in CSF • Enhancement remits spontaneously.

Imaging Signs

▶ **Modality of choice**
MRI.
▶ **CT findings**
Plain CT appears normal • Severe cases will show detectable meningeal enhancement.
▶ **MRI findings**
Findings on T1-weighted and T2-weighted images are normal • Severe cases will show detectable thickening of the dura mater on FLAIR images • Contrasted T1-weighted images show enhancement corresponding to the severity of irritation • Enhancement is invariably linear and not nodular • Only the dura mater is involved, never the leptomeninges • Leptomeningeal enhancement is invariably abnormal.

Clinical Aspects

▶ **Typical presentation**
Patients may be asymptomatic • Signs of post-lumbar puncture syndrome include headache, nausea, vomiting, and vertigo.
▶ **Treatment options**
Usually requires no treatment.
▶ **Course and prognosis**
Favorable prognosis.
▶ **What does the clinician want to know?**
Are these findings consistent with post-lumbar puncture syndrome?

Differential Diagnosis

Meningitis	– Differential diagnosis is not possible solely on the basis of imaging findings
	– Typical clinical findings with signs of inflammation in CSF
Spontaneous symptoms of reduced CSF pressure	– Post-lumbar puncture meningeal irritation may or may not belong in this category
	– Differential diagnosis on the basis of imaging findings is difficult
	– Enhancement can persist for months
	– Often occurs in association with subdural hematomas and hygromas

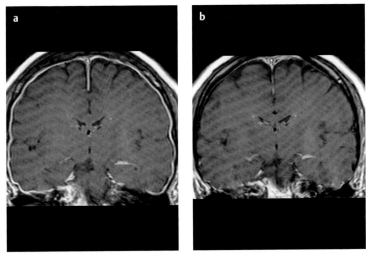

Fig. 8.3 a, b Coronal T1-weighted MR images after contrast administration three days (**a**) and fours weeks (**b**) after lumbar puncture. Significant enhancement of the dura mater several days after lumbar puncture (**a**). No meningeal enhancement is detected on the follow-up image four weeks later (**b**).

Tips and Pitfalls

Misinterpreting as meningitis.

Selected References

Hannerz J et al. MRI with gadolinium in patients with post-lumbar puncture headache. Acta Radiol 1999; 40 (2): 135–141

Krampla W et al. Lumbales meningeales Enhancement in der KM-MRT nach Operationen in der hinteren Schädelgrube. Eine normale Erscheinung bei Kindern. Rofo Fortschr Geb Rontgenstr Neuen Bildgeb Verfahr 2002; 174: 1511–1515

Thömke F et al. Spontanes Liquorunterdrucksyndrom. Klinische, neuroradiologische, nuklearmedizinische und Liquor-Befunde. Nervenarzt 1999; 70: 909–915

Definition

Epidemiology

Central nervous system involvement occurs in 10% of all cases of systemic sarcoidosis • *Incidence:* 0.02–0.05% • *Sex predilection:* Females • *Peak age:* 20–40 years.

Etiology, pathophysiology, pathogenesis

Systemic, granulomatous disorder with a tendency to perivascular spreading • Histology: granulomas with multinucleated giant cells and asteroid bodies are diagnostic • There are three basic patterns of CNS involvement: leptomeningeal, parenchymal, and vascular forms.

Imaging Signs

▶ **Modality of choice**
  MRI.

▶ **CT findings**
  Usually sharply demarcated lesions • Slightly hyperdense (hypodense lesions are the exception but do occur) • Homogeneously enhancing • Involvement of the hypothalamus, pituitary stalk, and base of the brain is characteristic • However, lesions can also occur diffusely throughout all parts of the brain.

▶ **MRI findings**
  Periventricular lesions • Hyperintense to brain tissue on T2-weighted and FLAIR images • Lesions on T1-weighted images are initially hypointense, and after enhancement are hyperintense for a long period • Perivascular spaces enhance • Cranial nerves (such as the facial and abducent nerves) enhance • Meningeal enhancement: en plaque or nodular pattern • Signs of basilar meningitis.

Clinical Aspects

▶ **Typical presentation**
  Cranial nerve palsy: facial and abducent nerves • Hypothalamic and pituitary dysfunction, occasionally with diabetes insipidus • Convulsions • Sensory deficits • Obstructed CSF flow (headache, vomiting, vertigo, papilledema) • Signs of meningeal irritation (headache, nausea, and vomiting).

▶ **Treatment options**
  Anti-inflammatory therapy, such as glucocorticoids.

▶ **Course and prognosis**
  Chronic courses may occur.

▶ **What does the clinician want to know?**
  Differentiate from neoplastic disorders • Localization • Extent.

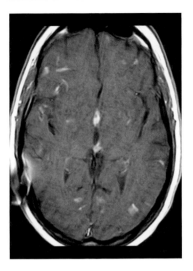

Fig. 8.4 CNS sarcoidosis. Axial T1-weighted MR image after contrast administration. Multifocal, nodular enhancing lesions. Enhancement in the basilar Virchow–Robin spaces.

Differential Diagnosis

Meningitis	– Perivascular spaces usually not involved – Usually no periventricular involvement
Meningioma en plaque	– No abnormal CSF findings – Slow course
Tuberculosis	– CSF findings – Differential diagnosis on the basis of imaging findings can be difficult in basilar meningitis
Lymphoma	– CSF findings – Usually no cranial nerve involvement – Other clinical course
Multiple sclerosis	– CSF findings, difficult differential diagnosis in the absence of basilar meningitis – Predilection for periventricular white matter – Lesions often in different stages (enhancement)

Fig. 8.5 Axial T1-weighted MR image after contrast administration, right cerebellopontine angle. Enhancement of the cranial nerves, a typical finding in CNS sarcoidosis. Enhancement of the nerve segment at the internal auditory canal (arrow) is consistent with unilateral facial nerve peripheral palsy.

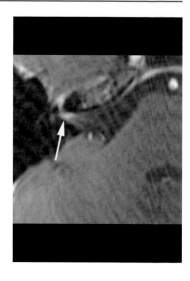

Tips and Pitfalls

Enhancement of the cranial nerves can persist for months despite abatement of clinical symptoms.

Selected References

Nowak DA et al. Neurosarcoidosis: a review of its intracranial manifestation. J Neurol 2001; 248: 363–372

Pickuth D et al. Wertigkeit der MRT in der Diagnostik der Neurosarkoidose. Radiologe 1999; 39: 889–893

Studler U et al. Basale Meningitis mit Hirnstamminsult bei Morbus Boeck. Rofo Fortschr Geb Rontgenstr Neuen Bildgeb Verfahr 2001; 173: 276–277

Woitalla D et al. Klinik und bildgebende Diagnostik der Sarkoidose des Nervensystems. Radiologe 2000; 40: 1064–1976

Definition

▶ **Etiology, pathophysiology, pathogenesis**

Imbalance between production and drainage or absorption of CSF.

Pathogenesis: Blockage of CSF drainage routes due to:

– Hemorrhage: Blood in the ventricles secondary to subarachnoid hemorrhage, cerebral hemorrhage that spreads to the ventricles, intraventricular hemorrhage.

– Mass: Colloid cysts at the interventricular foramen of Monro, obstruction of the foramen of Monro by extraventricular masses with midline displacement such as brain tumors.

– Other causes: Malignant cerebral infarctions (with mass effect), intraventricular tumor, choroid plexus papilloma, medulloblastoma, central neurocytoma.

– Stenosis of the cerebral aqueduct or the lateral and median apertures of the fourth ventricle due to external compression or idiopathic and/or postinflammatory changes: pineal cyst, choroid plexus papilloma, Chiari malformation (cerebral tonsils descended into the cervical canal) or malformations of the craniocervical junction.

Imaging Signs

▶ **Modality of choice**

– For diagnosis: CT and MRI.

– To determine the cause (except for cerebral hemorrhage): MRI.

▶ **CT and MRI findings**

CT and MRI: Enlarged ventricles • Increased intracranial pressure • Quotient of the distance between the frontal horns and the intracranial diameter (frontal horn index) > 0.33 • Width of the temporal horns > 3 mm • In acute hydrocephalus there will be a periventricular hypodensity on CT and hyperintensity on T2-weighted, proton density, and FLAIR images caused by CSF being forced through the ependyma.

Additional MRI findings: Thinning of the corpus callosum on sagittal images • Herniation of the third ventricle into the suprasellar cistern • Stenosis of the cerebral aqueduct appears as absence of fluid flow through the aqueduct on cine MRI and absence of a flow void on T2-weighted and proton density images.

Clinical Aspects

▶ **Typical presentation**

Headache • Optic disk edema • Nausea • Consciousness may be impaired.

▶ **Treatment options**

CSF shunt.

▶ **Course and prognosis**

Complications of a CSF shunt: subdural hygromas • Shunt infection • Slitlike ventricle • Shunt displacement.

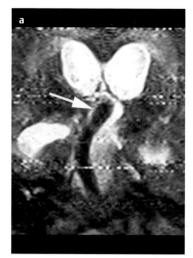 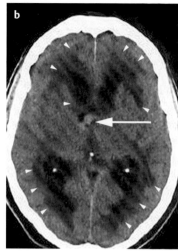

Fig. 9.1 a, b   Obstructive hydrocephalus. Coronal T2-weighted MR image (**a**) and axial CT (**b**). Enlarged lateral ventricles with CSF forced through the ependyma. Elongated basilar artery with cranial displacement of the floor of the third ventricle (**a, b**; arrows) and obstruction of the interventricular foramen; this causes lateral ventricular hydrocephalus with CSF forced through the ependyma (**b**; arrowheads).

Fig. 9.2   Sagittal T1-weighted MR image. Hydrocephalus from benign cerebral aqueduct stenosis with typical funnel-shaped proximal aqueduct (arrow).

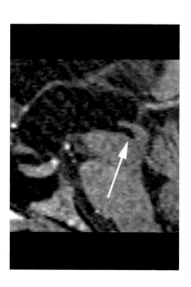

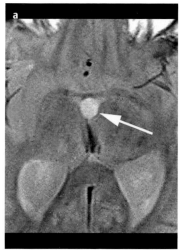 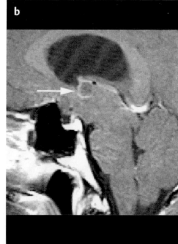

Fig. 9.3 a, b Axial proton density image (**a**) and sagittal T1-weighted MR image after IV contrast administration (**b**). Hydrocephalus due to colloid cyst (arrow) at the interventricular foramen of Monro.

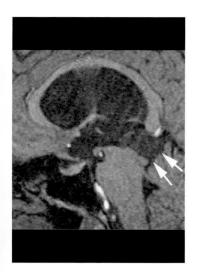

Fig. 9.4 Sagittal T1-weighted MR image. Hydrocephalus secondary to compression of the cerebral aqueduct by a pineal cyst (arrows).

▶ **What does the clinician want to know?**
Follow-up after shunting where obstructive hydrocephalus, idiopathic normal pressure hydrocephalus, or loss of brain volume has been diagnosed ● Signs of increased intracranial pressure.

Differential Diagnosis
....

Loss of brain volume	– Peripheral CSF spaces also enlarged
Idiopathic normal pressure hydrocephalus	– Typical clinical triad
	– Flow void in the cerebral aqueduct unlike findings in aqueduct stenosis

Selected References

Aronyk KE. The history and classification of hydrocephalus. Neurosurg Clin N Am 1993; 4 (4): 599–609

Mori K. Current concept of hydrocephalus: evolution of new classifications. Childs Nerv Syst 1995; 11 (9): 523–531; discussion 531–532

Definition

▶ **Epidemiology**
Usually diagnosed between the ages of 50 and 70 years ● Thirty to seventy percent of all cases represent secondary forms, such as may occur after subarachnoid hemorrhage.

▶ **Etiology, pathophysiology, pathogenesis**
Associated with vascular risk factors such as arterial hypertension, diabetes mellitus, heart disease, and arteriosclerosis ● Pathogenesis is not fully understood ● *Hypothesis:* Decreased compliance of the cerebral arteries due to ectasia, arteritis, spasm, microangiopathy, arachnoiditis, or posthemorrhagic adhesions ● There is insufficient physiologic attenuation of the wave of arterial pressure in the subarachnoid space ● The result is an increase in intracerebral pressure and the transcerebral brain mantle pressure gradient ● Pulsatile expansion of the brain occurs (primarily outward expansion) ● Chronic compression of the pontine veins ● Result: reduced cerebral blood flow.

Imaging Signs

▶ **Modality of choice**
MRI.

▶ **CT and MRI findings**
Symmetrical enlargement of the supratentorial inner CSF spaces without atrophy of the mantle of the brain ● Flattening of the gyri and narrowing of the peripheral CSF spaces above the margin of the brain mantle ● Basal cisterns and fourth ventricle appear normal ● Sixty percent of all cases are associated with medullar microangiopathy ● Accelerated CSF flow in the cerebral aqueduct.

Clinical Aspects

▶ **Typical presentation**
Typical triad of gait disturbance (unsteady, slowed, and irregular gait), bladder dysfunction (urge incontinence), and development of dementia with impaired memory, concentration, and drive ● Akinetic mutism occurs in rare cases.

▶ **Treatment options**
CSF drainage by shunting, possibly following removal of CSF via lumbar puncture.

▶ **Course and prognosis**
Findings improve postoperatively in 60–90% of patients ● Complete return to normal is rare ● The extent of postoperative improvement correlates negatively with the severity of the vascular encephalopathy.

▶ **What does the clinician want to know?**
Does the patient have idiopathic normal-pressure hydrocephalus, hydrocephalus due to other causes, or loss of brain volume?

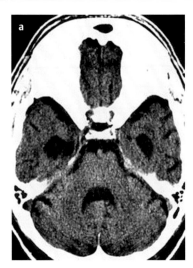

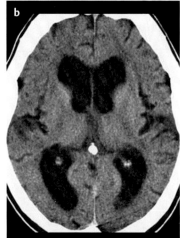

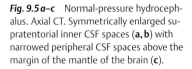

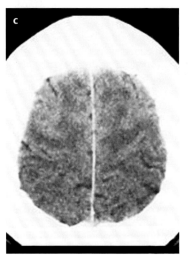

Fig. 9.5 a–c Normal-pressure hydrocephalus. Axial CT. Symmetrically enlarged supratentorial inner CSF spaces (**a, b**) with narrowed peripheral CSF spaces above the margin of the mantle of the brain (**c**).

Differential Diagnosis

Vascular dementia	– Multiple microangiopathic cerebral infarctions (Binswanger disease) or territorial (embolic) cerebral infarctions (multiple infarction dementia)
Obstructive hydrocephalus with stenosis of the cerebral aqueduct	– No detectable flow of the CSF in the aqueduct
Obstructive hydrocephalus from other causes	– Causes best visualized on MRI
Alzheimer disease	– Loss of volume of the medial temporal lobe, especially in the amygdala–hippocampus complex and the parahippocampal gyrus
Loss of brain volume	– Peripheral CSF spaces also enlarged

Tips and Pitfalls

Diagnosing idiopathic normal pressure hydrocephalus in the absence of an appropriate clinical context.

Selected References

Krauss JK et al. Vascular risk factors and arteriosclerotic disease in idiopathic normal-pressure hydrocephalus of the elderly. Stroke 1996; 27 (1): 24–29

Krauss JK et al. White matter lesions in patients with idiopathic normal pressure hydrocephalus and in an age-matched control group: a comparative study. Neurosurgery 1997; 40 (3): 491–495; discussion 495–496

Greitz D et al. The pathogenesis and hemodynamics of hydrocephalus. International Journal of Neuroradiology 1997; 3: 367–375

Gleason PL et al. The neurobiology of normal pressure hydrocephalus. Neurosurg Clin N Am 1993; 4 (4): 667–675

Definition

▶ **Etiology, pathophysiology, pathogenesis**
Synonym: Benign intracranial hypertension ● Significantly elevated CSF pressure ● CSF findings otherwise normal ● No detectable focal cerebral lesion.
Etiology is not known ● Usually occurs in obese women below age 30 years ● Incidence in obese women between the ages of 20 and 44 years is 19:100 000 per year.
Hypothesis: Obesity leads to elevated intra-abdominal pressure ● This in turn increases pleural pressure and cardiac filling pressure, impairing venous drainage in the brain.

Imaging Signs

▶ **Modality of choice**
MRI.
▶ **CT and MRI findings**
In 50–70% of cases, the enlarged suprasellar cisterns extend into the sellar region: The flattened pituitary gland lies on the floor of the sella turcica ("empty sella" sign) ● In 80% of cases, the globe is flattened at the point of entry of the optic nerve ● In 45% of cases, the CSF space is enlarged bilaterally around both optic nerves ● Occasionally, there is a slight Chiari I malformation ● Ventricular width is normal ● There are no abnormalities such as brain tumor, sinus thrombosis, or meningitis.

Clinical Aspects

▶ **Typical presentation**
Classic triad: Headache, impaired vision, papilledema ● Less often neck, back, and shoulder pain is also present.
▶ **Treatment options**
  – Treatment of the causes: Weight loss.
  – Symptomatic treatment for minor visual impairment: Acetazolamide (depresses CSF production), alternatively furosemide.
  – Severe or rapidly progressive visual impairment: Place head in elevated position and perform lumbar puncture with removal of CSF and osmotherapy.
  – Severe courses: Lumboperitoneal shunt and optic nerve sheath fenestration.
▶ **Course and prognosis**
Complications: Blindness occurs in 1% of cases ● Diminished visual acuity occurs in 10–20% of cases.
▶ **What does the clinician want to know?**
Radiologic signs of pseudotumor cerebri.

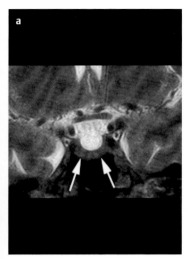
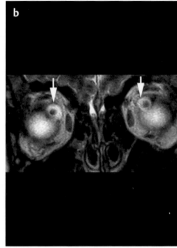

Fig. 9.6 a, b Pseudotumor cerebri. Coronal T2-weighted MR images (**a, b**). Flattened pituitary gland on the floor of the sella turcica (**a**; arrows). Bilateral enlargement of the CSF spaces around the optic nerves (**b**; arrows).

Differential Diagnosis

Secondary intracranial hypertension due to intracranial venous thrombosis, Addison disease, hyperparathyroidism, hypothyroidism, hematologic disease, collagen diseases, chronic encephalitis

- Acute or past intracranial venous thrombosis
- Hormone studies
- Encephalitic changes

Suprasellar arachnoid cyst

- Compression of the optic chiasm from below

Selected References

Friedman DI et al. Diagnostic criteria for idiopathic intracranial hypertension. Neurology 2002; 59 (10): 1492–1495

Wall M et al. Idiopathic intracranial hypertension. A prospective study of 50 patients. Brain 1991; 114 (Pt 1A): 155–180

Sugerman HJ et al. Increased intra-abdominal pressure and cardiac filling pressures in obesity-associated pseudotumor cerebri. Neurology 1997; 49 (2): 507–511

Definition

▶ **Etiology, pathophysiology, pathogenesis**
Usually caused by cerebral infarction ● Less often by tumors, hemorrhages, and vascular malformations.
Anterograde degeneration of a nerve fiber due to damage to the body of the nerve cell or its proximal axonal portions ● Most often detectable in the pyramidal tract, less often in the mamillothalamic tract, fornix, or corpus callosum.

Imaging Signs

▶ **Modality of choice**
MRI.
▶ **CT findings**
Often only volume loss of the affected areas in the terminal stage.
▶ **MRI findings**
  – Stage 1 (acute): For up to four weeks after the damage there is no signal abnormality on conventional MR images.
  – Stage 2 (subacute): After 4–14 weeks, T2-weighted images show hypointensity caused by initial physical but not biochemical breakdown of myelin and axon components.
  – Stage 3 (chronic): Hyperintensity on T2-weighted images (breakdown of fats and lipoproteins, vasogenic edema, gliosis).
  – Stage 4: Atrophy
  Early detection is possible with magnetization transfer (MT) technique and diffusion-weighted images.

Clinical Aspects

▶ **Typical presentation**
Depends on the primary disorder, such as stroke.
▶ **Treatment options**
No treatment is possible.
▶ **Course and prognosis**
Depends on the primary disorder.
▶ **What does the clinician want to know?**
Localization ● Extent ● Affected structures.

Differential Diagnosis

Two-stage cerebral infarction	– ADC is reduced in acute infarction
	– Does not extend only along tract structures but within an arterial territory
Cerebral edema	– Does not extend only along tract structures

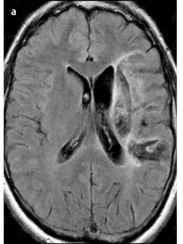

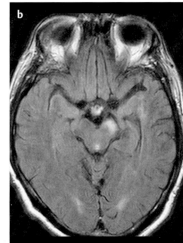

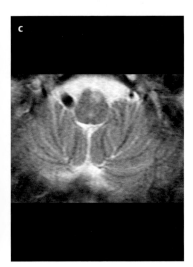

Fig. 10.1 a–c Wallerian degeneration secondary to middle cerebral artery infarction in the left cerebral hemisphere. Axial FLAIR images (**a, b**) and axial T2-weighted MR image (**c**). Cystic defect with gliosis in the territory of the left middle cerebral artery (**a**). Increased signal intensity in the pyramidal tract in the left cerebral peduncle (**b**) and left medulla oblongata (**c**).

Selected References

Castillo M et al. Early abnormalities related to postinfarction Wallerian degeneration: evaluation with MR diffusion-weighted imaging. J Comput Assist Tomogr 1999; 23 (6): 1004–1007

Yamada K et al. MR imaging of CNS tractopathy: wallerian and transneuronal degeneration. AJR Am J Roentgenol 1998; 171 (3): 813–818

Definition

▶ **Epidemiology**
The most common form of dementia ● *Frequency:* 8% in patients over 65 years ● Disorder of advanced age (age 60–90 years) ● Autosomal dominant familial Alzheimer begins between ages 30 and 40 years.

▶ **Etiology, pathophysiology, pathogenesis**
Shrinkage of the brain parenchyma, least severe in the occipital region ● Neuritic plaques in the hippocampus, neocortex, and subcortical region ● Loss of synapses and neurons ● Amyloid precursor protein plays a key role in the etiology of the disease ● In Alzheimer disease amyloid protein (Aβ) is the main component of the neuritic plaques and of the blood vessels ● In a separate process, Alzheimer fibrils (deposits of abnormal τ protein) develop in the cerebral cortex and basal ganglia.

Imaging Signs

▶ **Modality of choice**
MRI.

▶ **CT and MRI findings**
Loss of volume of the medial temporal lobe, especially in the amygdala–hippocampus complex and the parahippocampal gyrus.

Clinical Aspects

▶ **Typical presentation**
Initial symptoms include headache, vertigo, decreased cognitive facilities, depressive mood ● Later neurophysiologic deficits occur, including memory loss, and deficits in reading, writing, and arithmetic.

▶ **Treatment options**
Neuropsychologic training methods ● Compulsively restless patients are treated medically with neuroleptics.

▶ **Course and prognosis**
Slowly progressive ● Duration of the disorder until death is approximately 8–10 years.

▶ **What does the clinician want to know?**
Confirmation of the tentative diagnosis ● Exclude other forms of dementia.

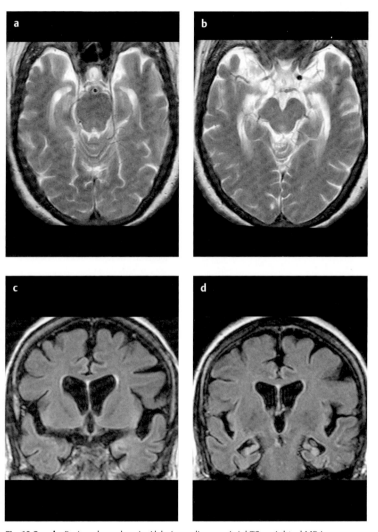

Fig. 10.2 a–d Brain volume loss in Alzheimer disease. Axial T2-weighted MR images (**a, b**) and coronal FLAIR images (**c, d**). Temporal and parietal cortical volume loss, especially in the hippocampus. Secondary enlargement of the temporal horns of the lateral ventricles.

Differential Diagnosis

Pick disease	– Cortical volume loss most pronounced in the fronto-temporal region and sparing the posterior two-thirds of the superior frontal gyrus
Normal-pressure hydrocephalus	– Typical clinical triad (dementia, gait disturbance, incontinence) – Widened infratentorial and supratentorial inner CSF spaces; peripheral CSF spaces are greatly narrowed or obliterated – Density and signal intensity abnormalities especially in the high frontoparietal periventricular and subcortical regions
Vascular dementia	– Multiple microangiopathic cerebral infarctions (Binswanger disease) or territorial embolic cerebral infarctions (multiple infarction dementia)
Creutzfeldt–Jakob disease	– Hyperintensity on FLAIR and T2-weighted MR images (reactive gliosis) and bilaterally reduced ADC (spongiform pathology) in the striatum (Creutzfeldt–Jakob disease) or bilaterally in the pulvinar of the thalamus (variant Creutzfeldt–Jakob disease)
Corticobasal degeneration	– Lenticular nucleus hypointense on T2-weighted MR images – Asymmetrical cortical volume loss
Progressive supranuclear palsy	– Volume loss in the midbrain – Hyperintensity of the mesencephalic tegmentum on T2-weighted MR images
Dementia associated with amyotrophic lateral sclerosis	– Hyperintensity of the internal capsule on T2-weighted MR images – Hypointensity of the cortex of the precentral gyrus on T2-weighted MR images
Huntington disease	– Volume loss of the head of the caudate nucleus
Wilson disease	– Hyperintensity or hypointensity of the lenticular nucleus on T2-weighted MR images

Selected References

Essig M et al. Radiologische Demenzdiagnostik. Radiologe 2003; 43 (7): 531–536

Hentschel F. Stellenwert der strukturellen und funktionellen Bildgebung bei Demenzen. Radiologie up2date 2004; 1: 37–56

Urbach H et al. Creutzfeldt-Jakob-Krankheit: Stellenwert der MRT. Röfo Fortschr Geb Röntgenstr Neuen Bildgeb Verfahr 2001; 173 (6): 509–514

Wenk GL. Neuropathologic changes in Alzheimer's disease. J Clin Psychiatry 2003; 64 (Suppl 9): 7–10

Definition

▶ **Etiology, pathophysiology, pathogenesis**
Alcoholism ● Malnutrition ● Cirrhosis of the liver ● Diabetes mellitus ● Derangements of electrolyte metabolism such as excessively rapid correction of hyponatremia ● Typical and most common form (50% of cases): central pontine myelinolysis ● In 10% of cases, extrapontine manifestation also occurs.

Imaging Signs

▶ **Modality of choice**
MRI.
▶ **CT findings**
Hypodensity in the affected areas.
▶ **MRI findings**
Symmetrical hyperintensity on T2-weighted images without apparent mass effect in the pons or at another site in the brain parenchyma, such as in the subcortical white matter, in the putamen, caudate nucleus, and midbrain.

Clinical Aspects

▶ **Typical presentation**
Disease is often biphasic:
– Initial symptoms include seizures and mental status changes.
– After a period of days or weeks: brainstem symptoms, impaired consciousness, impaired motion, pyramidal tract signs, tetraparesis, locked-in syndrome.
▶ **Treatment options**
Slower correction of electrolyte derangement ● Symptomatic treatment.
▶ **Course and prognosis**
Near total remission of symptoms occurs only in mild clinical courses
▶ **What does the clinician want to know?**
Extent of the pontine findings ● Extrapontine lesions.

Differential Diagnosis

Territorial pontine infarctions	– Wedge-shaped, usually unilateral
	– ADC invariably reduced initially
Pontine glioma	– Mass
Pontine microangiopathy	– Lesion not usually located only in the central pons
	– Changes also occur at another location in the brain parenchyma
	– ADC invariably increased

Fig. 10.3 Central pontine myelinolysis. Axial T2-weighted MR image. Symmetrical hyperintensity without apparent mass effect in the pons.

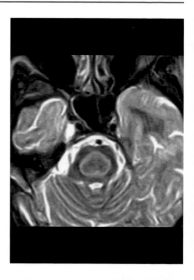

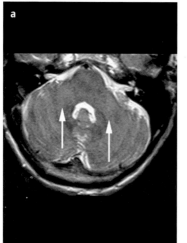

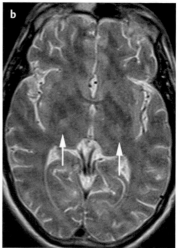

Fig. 10.4a, b Extrapontine myelinolysis in chronic recurrent hypoglycemia. Axial T2-weighted MR images. Slightly symmetrical hyperintensity without apparent mass in the middle cerebellar peduncles (**a**; arrows) and in the posterior crus of the internal capsule (**b**; arrows).

Tips and Pitfalls

Misinterpreting as a pontine tumor or pontine microangiopathy.

Selected References

Chu K et al. Diffusion-weighted MR findings of central pontine and extrapontine myelin-olysis. Acta Neurol Scand 2001; 104 (6): 385–388

Chua GC et al. MRI findings in osmotic myelinolysis. Clin Radiol 2002; 57 (9): 800–806

Cramer SC et al. Decreased diffusion in central pontine myelinolysis. AJNR Am J Neurora-diol 2001; 22 (8): 1476–1479

Laubenberger J et al. Central pontine myelinolysis: clinical presentation and radiologic findings. Eur Radiol 1996; 6 (2): 177–183

Definition

▶ **Etiology, pathophysiology, pathogenesis**
Causes: Endogenous and exogenous noxious agents such as ionizing radiation, cytostatic agents, drugs (alcohol, toluol, cocaine, heroin, amphetamines), environmental toxins, cyclosporin A.

 – Acute radiation injury: Edema appears while irradiation is still in progress ● Reversible ● Little prognostic significance.
 – Chronic radiation injury: Several months to 10 years ● Occurs in 70% of patients within two years of radiation therapy for brain tumor.
 – Focal radiation injury: Radiation necrosis.
 – Diffuse radiation injury: Radiation-induced demyelination with areas of diffuse gliosis.
 – Diffuse damage to the white matter from chemotherapy agents and drugs ● Cocaine and heroin also induce vasospastic ischemia with cerebral infarctions.
 – Encephalopathy induced by methotrexate or carmustine occurs in 10% of all patients treated intravenously with these drugs and 40% of patients treated intrathecally.
 – Leukoencephalopathy induced by cyclosporin A (in 4– 29% of patients treated with cyclosporin A): Probably a variant of hypertensive encephalopathy (hyperperfusion encephalopathy, reversible posterior encephalopathy).
 – Alcohol: Loss of volume in the cerebrum and cerebellum ● Unspecific multifocal damage to the white matter ● Central pontine or extrapontine myelinolysis ● Rarely, necrosis of the middle layers of the corpus callosum (Marchiafava–Bignami disease).

Imaging Signs

▶ **Modality of choice**
MRI.
▶ **CT and MRI findings**
Diffuse damage to the white matter: Affected areas show hypodensity (CT) and hyperintensity (T2-weighted and FLAIR images) ● They usually do not enhance.
Radiation necrosis: Lesion showing ring enhancement with pronounced perifocal edema in the irradiated field ● Lesser mass effect than a tumor ● rrCBV on MR perfusion images is at most 50% higher than in normal brain tissue.

Clinical Aspects

▶ **Typical presentation**
Early stage: Acute or subacute encephalopathy ● Oculomotor disturbance ● Mental status changes resulting from organic pathology.
▶ **Treatment options**
Elimination of the underlying cause insofar as this is possible.

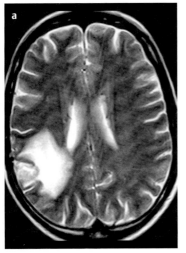 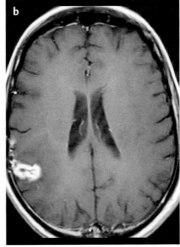

Fig. 10.5 a, b Radiation necrosis. Axial T2-weighted MR image (**a**) and axial T1-weighted MR image after contrast administration (**b**). Ring-enhancing structure (**b**) with a pronounced perifocal edema (**a**).

▶ **Course and prognosis**
Late sequelae: Mental status changes from organic brain disease ● Ataxia ● In severe cases, coma and death.

▶ **What does the clinician want to know?**
Differentiate from radiation necrosis, recurrent tumor, and abscess ● Extent of the lesions.

Differential Diagnosis
. . . .

Recurrent tumor	– Increased choline concentration on MRS
	– rrCBV on MR perfusion images twice as high as in normal brain tissue
	– Nuclear medicine studies (positron emission tomography with fluorine-18-deoxyglucose)
Cerebral abscess	– ADC reduced in cystic portion
	– No history of exposure to ionizing radiation
Hypertensive encephalopathy (hyperperfusion encephalopathy, reversible posterior encephalopathy)	– Pathology is usually reversible
ADEM (acute disseminated encephalomyelitis)	– Usually multiple lesions
	– No history of exposure to ionizing radiation

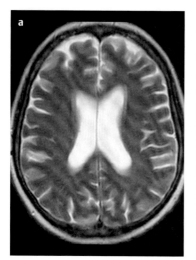 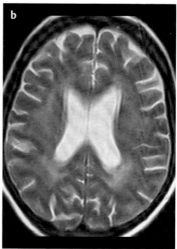

Fig. 10.6 a, b Diffuse radiation injury. Axial T2-weighted MR images. Prior to whole-brain irradiation for cerebellar metastasis of a breast carcinoma, the white matter of the centrum semiovale (**a**) shows a normal signal. Six months after whole-brain irradiation there are broad, diffuse hyperintensities consistent with radiation-induced demyelination with gliosis (**b**).

Tips and Pitfalls

Misinterpreting radiation necrosis as recurrent tumor.

Selected References

Cha S et al. Dynamic contrast-enhanced T2-weighted MR imaging of recurrent malignant gliomas treated with thalidomide and carboplatin. AJNR Am J Neuroradiol 2000; 21 (5): 881–90

Filley CM et al. Toxic leukoencephalopathy. N Engl J Med 2001; 345 (6): 425–32

Valk PE et al. Radiation injury of the brain. AJNR Am J Neuroradiol 1991; 12 (1): 45–62

Yamamoto A et al. CT and MRI findings of cyclosporine-related encephalopathy and hypertensive encephalopathy. Pediatr Radiol 2002; 32 (5): 340–343

Definition

▶ **Etiology, pathophysiology, pathogenesis**
Pathogenesis: Not known, presumably the result of reversibly increased permeability of the blood–brain barrier ● *Precipitating factors:* Hypertension or noxious agents, especially in the posterior cerebrovascular system where vascular autoregulation is not as efficient as in the area supplied by the anterior and middle cerebral arteries ● Occurs in patients with arterial hypertension but is not invariably associated with that disorder ● Associated with acute glomerulonephritis, preeclampsia, eclampsia, systemic lupus erythematosus, thrombotic thrombocytopenic purpura, hemolytic–uremic syndrome, drug toxicity (cyclosporin A, tacrolimus, cisplatin, erythropoietin).

Imaging Signs

▶ **Modality of choice**
MRI.
▶ **CT findings**
Symmetrical hypodensities in the posterior portions of the parietal and occipital lobes.
▶ **MRI findings**
Symmetrical hyperintensities (on T2-weighted and FLAIR images) and hypointensities (on T1-weighted images) in the parietal and occipital lobes ● Other rare localizations are frontal lobes, corpus callosum, brainstem, cerebellum, subcortical white matter and cerebral cortex ● Occasional subcortical enhancement ● Rarely hemorrhaging ● Changes are usually completely reversible ● Occasionally ADC is reduced, a sign of a cytotoxic cerebral edema; these lesions are usually irreversible.

Clinical Aspects

▶ **Typical presentation**
Headache ● Vertigo ● Vomiting ● Personality changes ● Seizures ● Arterial hypertension is not invariably present.
▶ **Treatment options**
Elimination of the noxious agent (control blood pressure, discontinue chemotherapy).
▶ **Course and prognosis**
Clinical and radiologic findings are usually reversible.
▶ **What does the clinician want to know?**
Differentiate from cerebral infarction and persistent toxic damage.

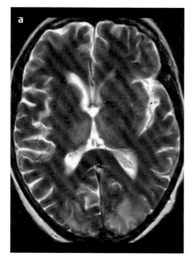

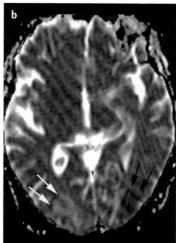

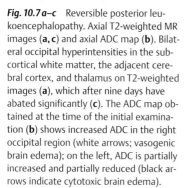

Fig. 10.7 a–c   Reversible posterior leukoencephalopathy. Axial T2-weighted MR images (**a, c**) and axial ADC map (**b**). Bilateral occipital hyperintensities in the subcortical white matter, the adjacent cerebral cortex, and thalamus on T2-weighted images (**a**), which after nine days have abated significantly (**c**). The ADC map obtained at the time of the initial examination (**b**) shows increased ADC in the right occipital region (white arrows; vasogenic brain edema); on the left, ADC is partially increased and partially reduced (black arrows indicate cytotoxic brain edema).

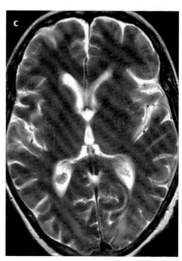

Differential Diagnosis

Embolic brain infarction	– Pattern of distribution corresponds to area supplied by one or more vessels
	– In acute stage ADC is invariably reduced
Toxic leukoencephalopathy	– Irreversible
Postictal transient cerebral hyperemia	– History of seizure
Progressive multifocal leuko-encephalopathy (PML)	– Only in immunocompromised persons

Tips and Pitfalls

Misinterpreting as a posterior cerebral artery infarction.

Selected References

Casey SO et al. Posterior reversible encephalopathy syndrome: utility of fluid-attenuated inversion recovery MR imaging in the detection of cortical and subcortical lesions. AJNR Am J Neuroradiol 2000; 21 (7): 1199–1206

Mukherjee P et al. Reversible posterior leukoencephalopathy syndrome: evaluation with diffusion-tensor MR imaging. Radiology 2001; 219 (3): 756–765

Provenzale JM et al. Quantitative assessment of diffusion abnormalities in posterior reversible encephalopathy syndrome. AJNR Am J Neuroradiol 2001; 22 (8): 1455–1461

Schilling S et al. MRI findings in acute hypertensive encephalopathy. Eur J Neurol 2003; 10 (3): 329–330

Leukoencephalopathies

Definition
....

▶ **Epidemiology**
Incidence: 0.6:100 000 per year ● Onset almost invariably above 35 years of age.

▶ **Etiology, pathophysiology, pathogenesis**
Multiple system neuronal degeneration with various clinical subtypes (striato-nigral degeneration, olivopontocerebellar atrophy, Shy–Drager syndrome, idio-pathic orthostatic hypotension) ● In the past, the subtypes were thought to be disorders from different causes ● Common neuropathologic feature: α-synu-clein-positive glial cytoplasmic inclusions in oligodendrocytes.

Imaging Signs
....

▶ **Modality of choice**
MRI.

▶ **MRI findings**
These findings occur in varying severity depending on the subtype:
– Volume loss in the pons and cerebellar peduncle, hemispheres, and vermis.
– Hyperintensities on T2-weighted and FLAIR images in the middle cerebellar peduncle.
– Atrophy and hypointensity on T2-weighted and T2*-weighted images in the putamen.
– Slit-shaped hypointensity on T2-weighted and T2*-weighted images lateral to the putamen.
– Reduced density of the pars compacta of the substantia nigra.
– Early signs: increased ADC in the putamen.

▶ **Nuclear medicine findings**
Changes in the glucose metabolism of the striatonigral system (PET) ● Changes in the striatonigral dopamine transport system (SPECT) ● Altered receptor bind-ing behavior in striatal iodobenzamide (SPECT) ● Cardiac sympathetic denerva-tion (scintigraphy).

Clinical Aspects
....

▶ **Typical presentation**
Autonomic and urogenital dysfunction ● Parkinson disease (bradykinesia, rigidi-ty, tremor) ● Cerebellar dysfunction (gait and extremity ataxia, ataxic dysarthria, nystagmus) ● Pyramidal tract signs.

▶ **Course and prognosis**
Mean survival time: 6–9 years.

▶ **Treatment options**
For Parkinson disease, levodopa, dopamine agonists, amantadine ● For ortho-static dysregulation, corticoids and sympathomimetics ● For focal dystonia, bot-ulinum toxin.

▶ **What does the clinician want to know?**
Demonstrate olivopontocerebellar or putaminal atrophy.

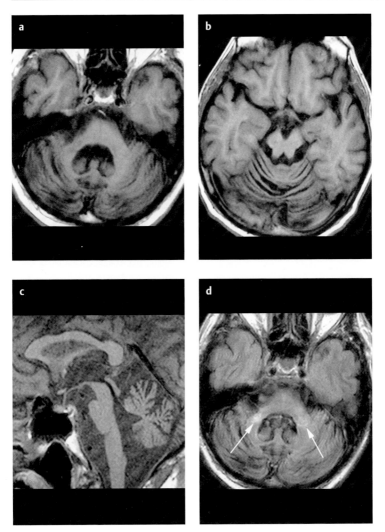

Fig. 10.8 a–d Multiple system atrophy. Axial T1-weighted MR images (**a**, **b**), sagittal T1-weighted MR image (**c**), and axial FLAIR image (**d**). Volume loss in the pons, cerebellum, and cerebellar peduncles (**a–c**). Hyperintensities in the middle cerebellar peduncles on the FLAIR image (**d**; arrows).

Differential Diagnosis

Paraneoplastic cerebellar degeneration	– Volume loss only in the cerebellum
Alcohol-induced volume loss	– Volume loss in the cerebrum as well

Selected References

Naka H et al. Characteristic MRI findings in multiple system atrophy: comparison of the three subtypes. Neuroradiology 2002; 44 (3): 204–209

Wenning GK et al. Multiple system atrophy. Lancet Neurol 2004; 3 (2): 93–103

Definition

▶ **Etiology, pathophysiology, pathogenesis**
Autosomal recessive metabolic disorder ● Insufficient excretion of copper in gall (due to lack of ceruloplasmin) ● Copper deposits excessively in many tissues, especially in the liver and brain (primarily in the basal ganglia) ● This results in impaired activity of various enzymes or cell destruction.

Imaging Signs

▶ **Modality of choice**
MRI.
▶ **CT findings**
Often negative ● Hypodensity in the caudate nucleus ● Rarely loss of brain volume ● Rarely hyperdensity in the putamen (deposits of iron and copper).
▶ **MRI findings**
Hyperintensity (T2-weighted, proton density, and FLAIR images) or hypointensity (T1-weighted images) consistent with cystic or necrotic changes due to loss of neurons in the affected structures (putamen, thalamus, caudate nucleus, red nucleus, superior cerebellar peduncle; less often in the subcortical white matter, gray matter around the cerebral aqueduct, pallidum, dentate nucleus) ● The putamen usually also exhibits a central hypointensity (on T2-weighted, proton density, and T2*-weighted images) from iron and copper deposits ● Rarely loss of brain volume ● Lesions are occasionally reversible under therapy.

Clinical Aspects

▶ **Typical presentation**
Depending on the pattern and severity of involvement: ● Dystonia ● Bradykinesia ● Hyperreflexia ● Dysdiadochokinesia ● Unsteadiness of gait ● Dysarthria ● Cranial nerve and gaze palsy ● Nystagmus ● Ataxia or asymptomatic condition ● Corneal pigment ring (Kayser–Fleischer ring).
▶ **Treatment options**
Symptomatic treatment of the disturbed copper metabolism.
▶ **Course and prognosis**
Good with early onset of treatment ● Fatal if left untreated.
▶ **What does the clinician want to know?**
Confirm the tentative diagnosis.

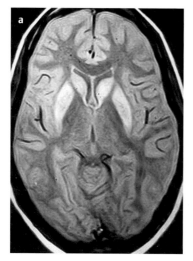

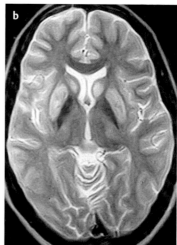

Fig. 10.9 a–c Axial proton density-weighted MR image (**a**) and axial T2-weighted MR images (**b, c**). Hyperintensity in the putamen and in the caudate nucleus (**a, b**). Hypointensity is also seen in the pallidum and red nucleus on T2-weighted images (**b, c**).

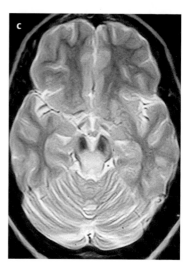

Differential Diagnosis

Venous infarction	– Intracranial venous thrombosis is usually also present – Occurs within a venous territory
Hypoxic–ischemic encephalopathy	– History of cardiopulmonary resuscitation or other such cardiovascular event – Involvement is not limited to basal ganglia – Within a few days, demarcation resembles ischemic cerebral infarction
Toxic encephalopathy	– Involvement is not limited to basal ganglia – Pathology is often reversible

Selected References

Magalhaes AC et al. Wilson's disease: MRI with clinical correlation. Neuroradiology 1994; 36 (2): 97–100

Definition

▶ **Etiology, pathophysiology, pathogenesis**
Often associated with alcoholic liver cirrhosis, chronic hepatitis, and portosystemic shunt • Chronic hepatic insufficiency leads to inadequate detoxification of neurotoxins such as ammonia, mercaptans, phenols, and short-chain fatty acids • Impaired excretion of manganese in the gall • Compromised blood–brain barrier leads to accumulation of neurotoxins and deposits of manganese in the basal ganglia and at other sites • Alzheimer type II astrocyte gliosis in the areas with manganese deposits.

Imaging Signs

▶ **Modality of choice**
MRI.
▶ **CT findings**
No typical findings.
▶ **MRI findings**
T1-weighted images show bilateral symmetrical hyperintensities in the basal ganglia, rarely also in the caudate nucleus, subthalamic nucleus, and pituitary (deposits of paramagnetic manganese) • The extent of basal ganglion pathology correlates with the level of plasma ammonia and neurologic deficits • Similar findings occur in prolonged parenteral feeding and in persons exposed to manganese.

Clinical Aspects

▶ **Typical presentation**
Slight neuropsychologic deficits • Sleep disturbances • Restlessness • Personality changes • Disorientation and loss of consciousness occur in later stages of the disorder.
▶ **Treatment options**
Treatment of the liver disorder.
▶ **Course and prognosis**
This depends on the underlying disorder.
▶ **What does the clinician want to know?**
Differentiation from other basal ganglion pathology such as calcifications.

Differential Diagnosis

Neurofibromatosis type I	– Other neuroradiologic and clinical signs of neurofibromatosis type I
Fine, disseminated calcifications with high signal intensity on T1-weighted MR images	– Definitively demonstrated on CT

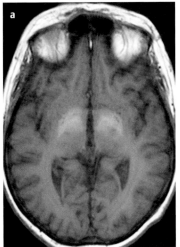 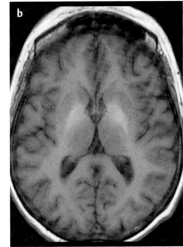

Fig. 10.10 a, b Hepatic encephalopathy. Noncontrasted T1-weighted MR images. Bilateral symmetrical hyperintensities in the basal ganglia.

Selected References

Kulisevsky J et al. Magnetic resonance imaging pallidal hypersignal in cirrhotic subjects. Hepatology 1996; 24 (1): 282–283

Lockwood AH. Hepatic encephalopathy. Neurol Clin 2002; 20 (1): 241–246

Lucchini R et al. Brain magnetic resonance imaging and manganese exposure. Neurotoxicology 2000; 21 (5): 769–775

Definition

▶ **Epidemiology**
The most common neurologic systemic disorder • *Frequency:* 1.8:100000 • *Mean age of occurrence:* 65 years.

▶ **Etiology, pathophysiology, pathogenesis**
Etiology is unclear • Sometimes occurs as paraneoplasia • Severe, chronic degenerative disorder of the central nervous system • Primarily involves the motor system • *Pathology:* Loss of pyramidal cells in the motor cortex with gliosis in layers II and III • Subsequent degeneration of the motor pathway (first and second motor neurons) • Atrophy of the anterior spinal nerve roots.

Imaging Signs

▶ **Modality of choice**
MRI.

▶ **CT findings**
Cortical atrophy, often in the precentral gyrus.

▶ **MRI findings**
Cortical atrophy (precentral gyrus; parietal, insular, frontal, temporal cortex) • Low signal in the cortex of the precentral gyrus on T2-weighted images (increased iron deposits) • Increased signal in the pyramidal tract on T2-weighted, proton density, and FLAIR images, not only in the posterior crus of the internal capsule as occasionally occurs in normal persons but extending into the cerebral peduncles and the corona radiata (detectable in 78% of patients with rapidly progressive disease and in 12% of patients with slowly progressive disease) • Occasionally there is a signal increase in the cervical spinal cord as well.
Diffusion tensor imaging: Fractional anisotropy is reduced in the pyramidal tract, corpus callosum, and thalamus even before the onset of clinical symptoms.
MR spectroscopy: Loss of *N*-acetylaspartate (neuron marker).

Clinical Aspects

▶ **Typical presentation**
Progressive muscle weakness and atrophy • Combination of atrophic and spastic paralysis • No mental status changes • Bulbar paralysis occurs in 20% of cases.

▶ **Treatment options**
Physical therapy • Anabolic steroids • Anticonvulsants • Atropine preparations as well where bulbar symptoms are present.

▶ **Course and prognosis**
Mean duration of the disease until death: 25 months • Only one-third of all patients live longer than five years after the onset of disease.

▶ **What does the clinician want to know?**
Exclude other disorders • Confirm the tentative diagnosis (possible only in a few of the patients).

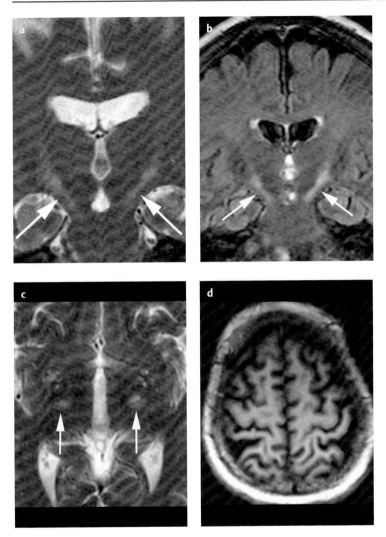

Fig. 10.11 a–d Amyotrophic lateral sclerosis. Coronal T2-weighted MR image (**a**), coronal FLAIR image (**b**), and axial T2-weighted MR image (**c**). Typical bilateral hyperintensities along the pyramidal tract (arrows). Atrophy of the precentral and postcentral gyri (**d**).

Differential Diagnosis

Normal pyramidal tract signal increase in the posterior crus of the internal capsule on T2-weighted MR images (detectable in 50% of the normal population)	– Signal increase more punctate
Multiple sclerosis	– Focal hyperintensities in the periventricular white matter and corpus callosum in the brainstem, and/or in the midbrain and cerebellum. – Nodular or ring enhancement may occur (McDonald criteria with dissemination over space and time)
Cervical myelopathy in cervical spinal stenosis	– Focal myelopathy signal at the level of the spinal stenosis
Syringomyelia	– Cavity in the spinal cord isointense to CSF
Spinal cord tumor	– Mass effect and enhancement

Tips and Pitfalls

Overlooking other radiologically detectable organic changes that would explain the clinical symptoms (El Escorial criteria):
– Bony changes in the skull or spine.
– Intraparenchymal or extraparenchymal processes in the brain or spinal cord such as tumors, inflammation, or vascular malformations.

Selected References

Comi G et al. Review neuroimaging in amyotrophic lateral sclerosis. Eur J Neurol 1999; 6 (6): 629–637

Sach M et al. Diffusion tensor MRI of early upper motor neuron involvement in amyotrophic lateral sclerosis. Brain 2004; 127 (Pt 2): 340–350

Definition

▶ **Etiology, pathophysiology, pathogenesis**
Vitamin B_1 (thiamine) deficiency ● Common in alcoholism, stomach disorders, hyperemesis, cirrhosis of the liver, malignant tumors, and pregnancy.

Imaging Signs

▶ **Modality of choice**
MRI.
▶ **CT findings**
Usually negative.
▶ **MRI findings**
Typical topographic distribution (periventricular regions) ● Hyperintensities on T2-weighted, proton density, and FLAIR images at these sites:
– Medial thalamic nuclei.
– Interthalamic adhesion.
– Floor of the third ventricle.
– Mamillary bodies.
– Reticular formation.
– Mesencephalic tectum and gray matter around the cerebral aqueduct.
Affected structures may enhance ● There may be petechial hemorrhages in the affected structures (hyperintensity on noncontrasted T1-weighted images) ● Chronic cases show enlargement of the third ventricle and volume loss in the mammillary bodies.

Clinical Aspects

▶ **Typical presentation**
Acute or subacute encephalopathy with oculomotor disturbances and psycho-physiologic changes occur in the early stage ● Later, mental status changes resulting from organic brain disease and ataxia.
▶ **Treatment options**
Early sufficient substitution of vitamin B_1.
▶ **Course and prognosis**
Invariably fatal if left untreated ● Death occurs in 10–20% of cases even with treatment ● Permanent organic psychologic syndrome persists in 80% of the survivors.
▶ **What does the clinician want to know?**
Confirm and ascertain the extent of findings.

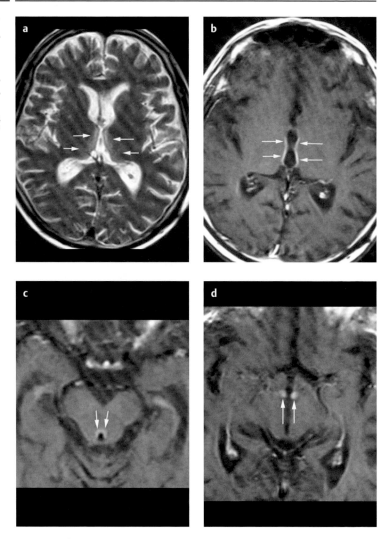

Fig. 10.12 a–d   Wernicke encephalopathy. Axial T2-weighted MR image (**a**) and axial T1-weighted MR images (**b–d**) after IV contrast administration. Typical signal increases in the medial thalamic nuclei on the T2-weighted image (**a**; arrows) with enhancement (**b**; arrows). Enhancement is also seen in the gray matter around the cerebral aqueduct (**c**; arrows) and in the mamillary bodies (**d**; arrows).

Leukoencephalopathies

Differential Diagnosis
....

Atypical primary intracerebral lymphoma with ependymal growth	– Ependymal enhancement is less symmetrical and often nodular

Selected References

Weidauer S et al. Wernicke encephalopathy: MR findings and clinical presentation. Eur Radiol 2003; 13 (5): 1001–1009

Definition

▶ **Etiology, pathophysiology, pathogenesis**
Hemosiderin deposits on the surface of the cerebrum, cerebellum, brainstem, spinal cord, or cranial nerves ● *Sequela:* Gliosis, loss of neurons and demyelination ● *Causes:* History of subarachnoid hemorrhage, often secondary to removal of ependymomas or other tumors of the posterior cranial fossa ● Hemosiderin-filled macrophages often remain behind after breaking down hemoglobin to hemosiderin ● A metabolic defect similar to hemochromatosis may also be present ● Cause remains unclear in 40% of cases.

Imaging Signs

▶ **Modality of choice**
MRI.
▶ **CT findings**
Usually normal; lesions are often incidental findings ● There may be slight hyperdensity on the surface of the brainstem.
▶ **MRI findings**
Hypointense halo on the surface of the cerebrum, cerebellum, brainstem, spinal cord, or cranial nerves on T2-weighted images ● There may be volume loss in the cerebellum.

Clinical Aspects

▶ **Typical presentation**
Dysarthria ● Progressive cerebellar ataxia in 88% of cases ● Sensorineural hearing loss in 95% of cases ● Neuropsychologic abnormalities ● MRI findings may precede clinical presentation and are not necessarily related to symptoms.
▶ **Treatment options**
Elimination of the underlying disorder ● Radical-binding agents (vitamins C and E) or chelating agents.
▶ **Course and prognosis**
Findings persist.
▶ **What does the clinician want to know?**
Cause ● Extent of findings.

Differential Diagnosis

Chemical shift artifacts	– No history of subarachnoid hemorrhage
	– Artifacts are not limited to the surface of the brain but also appear at other sites

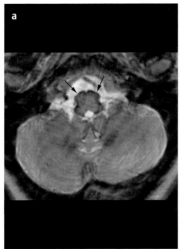

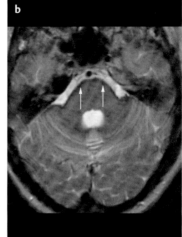

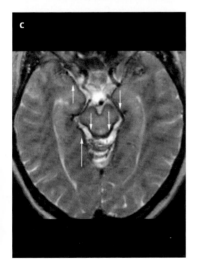

Fig. 10.13 a–c Superficial siderosis of the brain. Axial T2-weighted MR images. Hypointense halo (arrows) on the surface of the medulla oblongata and pons (**a, b**), midbrain (**c**), and medial temporal lobe (**c**).

Selected References

Fearnley JM et al. Superficial siderosis of the central nervous system. Brain 1995; 118 (Pt 4): 1051–1066

Leussink VI et al. Superficial siderosis of the central nervous system: pathogenetic heterogeneity and therapeutic approaches. Acta Neurol Scand 2003; 107 (1): 54–61

Congenital Malformations

Definition

▶ **Etiology, pathophysiology, pathogenesis**
Primary neurulation disturbance (defective closure of the neural tube) in the fourth to fifth weeks of pregnancy.
Chiari I malformation: Slight incongruity between the posterior cranial fossa (slightly too small) and the cerebellum (normal size), resulting in low-lying cerebellar tonsils • Associated malformations: hydrocephalus, syringomyelia, skeletal anomalies (basilar invagination, Klippel–Feil syndrome, atlantoaxial fusion).
Arnold–Chiari malformation (Chiari II malformation): Complex anomaly with skull, dural, brain, spinal, and spinal cord manifestations • Associated malformations: almost invariably lumbar myelomeningocele, syringomyelia (50–90%), diastematomyelia, anomalies of the corpus callosum, heterotopia.
Chiari III malformation: Arnold–Chiari malformation with deep occipital or high cervical encephalocele with cerebellar herniation.

Imaging Signs

▶ **Modality of choice**
MRI.

Chiari I Malformation

▶ **CT findings**
Abnormally high quantity of brain tissue in the foramen magnum • There may be ventricular enlargement • Narrowed peripheral CSF spaces above the surface of the cerebellum.

▶ **MRI findings**
Triangular tonsils • Narrowed peripheral CSF spaces above the surface of the cerebellum • Low-lying cerebellar tonsils, more than 5 mm below the level of the foramen magnum (opisthion–basion line) • Syringomyelia in 20–40% of all patients • Reduced CSF flow in the foramen magnum.

Arnold–Chiari Malformation (Chiari II Malformation)

▶ **CT findings**
Calvarial defects • Concave clivus.

▶ **MRI findings**
Extreme elongation of the cerebellar tonsils, which can extend to the level of the C4 vertebra • Elongated fourth ventricle • Beak-shaped tectum • Z-shaped kink at the junction of the medulla oblongata and cervical spinal cord • Interdigitation of the gyri of the cerebral hemispheres • Cerebellum is pressed against the brainstem and bulges superiorly past the tentorial notch • Hydrocephalus • Large interthalamic adhesion • Fenestrated flax cerebri • Low-lying transverse sinus and confluence of sinuses • Narrowed posterior cranial fossa, concave clivus.

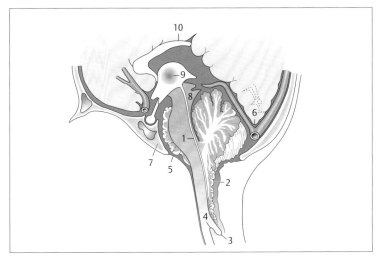

Fig. 11.1 Schematic diagram of the pathology in Arnold–Chiari malformation (1 = elongated fourth ventricle; 2 = pronounced elongation of the cerebellar tonsils displaced into the spinal canal; 3 = spinal cord "spurs" 4 = spinal cord kink; 5 = cerebellum pressed against the brainstem; 6 = low-lying confluence of the sinuses; 7 = concave clivus; 8 = beak-shaped tectum; 9 = large interthalamic adhesion; 10 = partial agenesis of the corpus callosum).

Clinical Aspects

▶ **Typical presentation/Course and prognosis**
  Chiari I malformation: Fifty percent of all cases are asymptomatic ● Brainstem compression produces cranial nerve dysfunction ● Somnolence ● Neck pain ● Symptomatic syringomyelia can imitate the clinical picture of multiple sclerosis.
  Arnold–Chiari malformation (Chiari II malformation): Myelomeningocele ● Macrocephaly ● Sphincter weakness ● Bulbar signs ● Elevated α-fetoprotein.
▶ **Treatment options**
  Treatment of myelomeningocele or hydrocephalus where present ● Decompressive osteotomy of the foramen magnum.
▶ **What does the clinician want to know?**
  Follow-up with hydrocephalus ● Demonstrate associated malformations such as myelomeningocele.

Fig. 11.2 Chiari I malformation. Sagittal T1-weighted MR image. Low-lying cerebellar tonsils, approximately 10 mm lower than the foramen magnum, are the only abnormal findings.

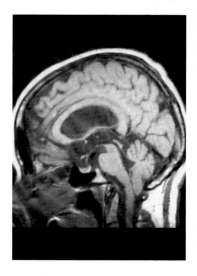

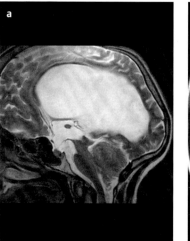

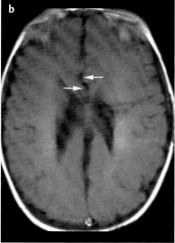

Fig. 11.3 a, b Arnold–Chiari (Chiari II) malformation. Sagittal T2-weighted MR image (**a**) and axial T1-weighted MR image (**b**). Beak-shaped tectum, hydrocephalus, and a narrowed posterior cranial fossa (**a**). Meshing of the gyri (**b**; arrows).

Differential Diagnosis

Acquired low-lying cerebellar tonsils in the presence of basilar impression or elevated intracranial pressure	– Basilar impression – Elevated intracranial pressure
Hydrocephalus from other causes	– Demonstrate the cause, best done with MRI

Selected References

McLone DG et al. The Chiari II malformation: cause and impact. Childs Nerv Syst 2003; 19 (7–8): 540–550

Naidich TP et al. Computed tomographic signs of the Chiari II malformation. Part I: Skull and dural partitions. Radiology 1980; 134 (1): 65–71

Shuman RM. The Chiari malformations: a constellation of anomalies. Semin Pediatr Neurol 1995; 2 (3): 220–226

Definition

▶ **Etiology, pathophysiology, pathogenesis**
Form of secondary neurulation disturbance (defective cellular migration) in the second to fifth months of pregnancy ● This results in collections of neurons in abnormal locations ● *Cause:* Cessation of radial migration of the neuroblasts.
Three groups are differentiated:
  – Subependymal heterotopias.
  – Focal subcortical heterotopias.
  – Diffuse heterotopias (band heterotopias, "double cortex").

Imaging Signs

▶ **Modality of choice**
MRI.
▶ **MRI findings**
Nodular or broad subependymal, periventricular, or subcortical regions that are isointense to gray matter on T1-weighted and T2-weighted images ● No perifocal edema ● No enhancement ● Best demonstrated on T1-weighted inversion recovery images.
Subependymal heterotopia: Oval structures with smooth margins that appear to dent the walls of the lateral ventricles.
Focal subcortical heterotopia: Areas of cortical infolding resembling vascular structures.
Diffuse heterotopia (band heterotopia, "double cortex"): Ribbon of gray matter deep to the cerebral cortex and separated from the cortex by a layer of white matter that appears normal ● The cerebral cortex lying above that layer can be normal or dysplastic (pachygyric) ● The thickness of the heterotopic gray matter correlates with the severity of the dysplasia of the overlying cortex.

Clinical Aspects

▶ **Typical presentation/Course and prognosis**
All forms are almost invariably associated with seizures.
Diffuse heterotopia: Moderate to severe developmental anomalies.
Focal subcortical heterotopia: Variable motor and intellectual disturbances.
Subependymal heterotopia: Intellectual and motor development usually normal ● Epileptic seizures begin at age 10 years.
▶ **Treatment options**
Symptomatic treatment of seizures.
▶ **What does the clinician want to know?**
Classify the heterotopia (differentiate focal from diffuse) ● Look for the focus in epilepsy.

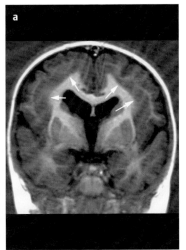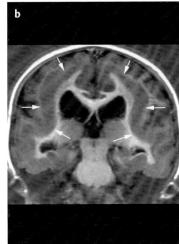

Fig. 11.4 a, b Diffuse heterotopia (band heterotopia, "double cortex"). Coronal T1-weighted MR images. Bandlike structure lying deep to the cortex (arrows), with a signal isointense to gray matter. A narrow band of normal white matter is visualized between the heterotopia and the cortex.

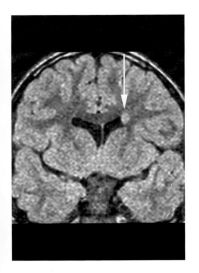

Fig. 11.5 Subependymal heterotopia. Coronal FLAIR image. Smoothly demarcated nodule isointense to gray matter that appears to dent the walls of the lateral ventricles (arrow).

Differential Diagnosis

Brain tumors	– Perifocal edema often present
	– Occasionally enhance
Cortical dysplasia	– Invariably in the cortex
	– Blurred demarcation between gray and white matter
Hamartomas in tuberous sclerosis	– Isointense to hyperintense to mature white matter
	– Not isointense to gray matter

Tips and Pitfalls

Failing to obtain high-resolution images with good contrast between gray and white matter.

Selected References

Barkovich AJ. Magnetic resonance imaging: role in the understanding of cerebral malformations. Brain Dev 2002; 24 (1): 2–12

D'Incerti L. Morphological neuroimaging of malformations of cortical development. Epileptic Disord 2003; 5 [Suppl 2]: S59-S-66

Congenital Malformations

Definition

▶ **Etiology, pathophysiology, pathogenesis**
Form of secondary neurulation disturbance (defect of cellular migration) in the second to fifth months of pregnancy • Development of the corpus callosum from anterior to posterior: first rostrum, then genu, then truncus, and lastly splenium. *Associated malformations:* Arnold–Chiari malformation • Defective migration • Encephaloceles • Dandy–Walker malformation • Holoprosencephaly • Azygos anterior cerebral artery • Midline lipomas.

Imaging Signs

▶ **Modality of choice**
MRI.
▶ **CT and MRI findings**
High third ventricle opening superiorly into the longitudinal fissure • Parallel, nonconverging lateral ventricles • Longitudinal fibers of white matter (Probst bundles) impress the middle margins of the superomedial portions of the lateral ventricles, giving the ventricles a half-moon shape • Radial orientation of the gyri • Colpocephaly (disproportionate enlargement of the occipital horns of the lateral ventricles).

Clinical Aspects

▶ **Typical presentation/Course and prognosis**
Seizures • Retarded development • Microencephaly • Hypertelorism • Hypothalamic and/or pituitary dysfunction.
▶ **Treatment options**
Symptomatic treatment of seizures and/or hypothalamic/pituitary dysfunction.
▶ **What does the clinician want to know?**
Associated malformations?

Differential Diagnosis

Secondary damage to the corpus callosum	– Complete but hypoplastic corpus callosum or absence of only the anterior portions
Semilobar holoprosencephaly	– Truncus of the corpus callosum is absent; a rudimentary splenium is present

Tips and Pitfalls

Failing to obtain sagittal T1-weighted MR images • Misinterpreting as hydrocephalus from a different cause.

Selected References

Barkovich AJ. Magnetic resonance imaging: role in the understanding of cerebral malformations. Brain Dev 2002; 24 (1): 2–12

Congenital Malformations

Fig. 11.6 Agenesis of the corpus callosum. Sagittal T1-weighted MR image.

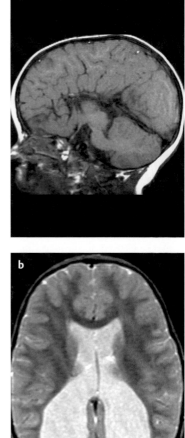

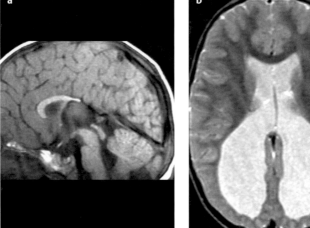

Fig. 11.7 a, b Dysgenesis of the corpus callosum. Sagittal T1-weighted MR image (**a**) and axial T2-weighted MR image (**b**). Hypoplasia of the posterior corpus callosum (parts of the truncus and splenium) with normally developed rostrum and genu (**a, b**). Colpocephaly (bilateral enlargement of the posterior horns of the lateral ventricles).

Congenital Malformations

Definition

▶ **Etiology, pathophysiology, pathogenesis**
Form of secondary neurulation disturbance (defective ventral induction) in the fifth to tenth weeks of pregnancy ● Dandy–Walker malformation and Dandy–Walker variant together form the Dandy–Walker complex.
Localization of the malformations: Skull and dura mater ● Ventricles and posterior cranial fossa ● Cerebellar hemispheres ● Cerebellar vermis ● Brainstem.
Associated malformations: Hypogenesis of the corpus callosum (30% of cases) ● Microgyria (polymicrogyria) or heterotopia of the gray matter (5–10%) ● Occipital encephalocele (16%) ● Schizencephaly ● Sacrolumbar meningocele.

Imaging Signs

▶ **Modality of choice**
MRI.
▶ **MRI findings**
Dandy–Walker malformation: Large posterior cranial fossa ● The rudimentary tentorium cerebelli, transverse sinus, and confluence of the sinuses are displaced cranially ● Hypogenesis or agenesis of the cerebellar vermis ● Cystic enlargement of the fourth ventricle, which extends posteriorly to between the widely spaced cerebellar hemispheres ● In 80% of cases there is obstructive hydrocephalus.
Dandy–Walker variant: Hypogenesis of the cerebellar vermis ● Cystic enlargement of the fourth ventricle which communicates through a narrow aperture with the subarachnoid space ("keyhole" deformity) ● There is no enlargement of the posterior cranial fossa.

Clinical Aspects

▶ **Typical presentation/Course and prognosis**
Retarded development ● Depends on the severity of the hydrocephalus and possible additional supratentorial malformations ● Seizures ● Impaired vision and hearing ● Hydrocephalus with protrusion of the occiput is present in 75% of all patients at the age of 3 months.
▶ **Treatment options**
Treatment of the hydrocephalus and seizures.
▶ **What does the clinician want to know?**
Differentiate from mega-cisterna magna and arachnoid cyst ● Follow-up studies of hydrocephalus.

Congenital Malformations

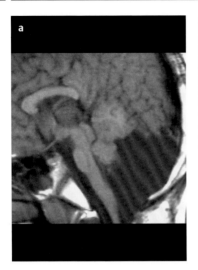
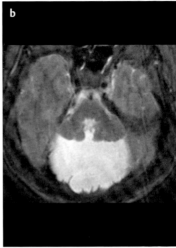

Fig. 11.8 a, b   Dandy–Walker malformation. Sagittal T1-weighted MR image (**a**) and axial T2-weighted MR image (**b**). Large posterior cranial fossa. Agenesis of the cerebellar vermis and cystic enlargement of the fourth ventricle, which extends posteriorly to between the widely spaced cerebellar hemispheres.

Differential Diagnosis

Mega-cisterna magna	– Enlargement of the posterior cranial fossa – Large cisterna magna with normal cerebellar vermis and normal fourth ventricle
Arachnoid cyst	– Cerebellum shows normal development – Fourth ventricle and cerebellar vermis may be displaced – Skull is often thinned – Often intrathecal contrast administration is required to differentiate from mega-cisterna magna as arachnoid cysts and mega-cisterna magna are isointense to CSF

Tips and Pitfalls

Misinterpreting mega-cisterna magna or arachnoid cyst as Dandy–Walker complex.

Selected References

ten Donkelaar HJ et al. Development and developmental disorders of the human cerebellum. J Neurol 2003; 250 (9): 1025–1036

Definition

▶ **Epidemiology**
The disorder affects 85% of newborns with a birth weight between 990 g and 2200 g who survive longer than six days.

▶ **Etiology, pathophysiology, pathogenesis**
The pathogenetic mechanisms and pathologic picture depend on the time of the damage:

- Premature newborns: Hypoxic brain damage in premature newborns ● Germinal matrix ischemia or hemorrhage.
- Term newborns: During the third trimester, the intervascular boundary zones, or "watershed," migrate from the subependymal (paramedian) region to the parasagittal region ● Parasagittal medullary damage in term newborns then occurs.
- Damage to the brain prior to the sixth month of pregnancy: Liquefaction of tissue necrosis with formation of cysts without residual gliosis ● Incorporation of the cysts into the lateral ventricles within 2–6 weeks.
- Damage to the brain beginning in the seventh month of pregnancy: Residual gliosis in addition to other findings (reactive astrocyte gliosis).

Typical localization: White matter around the posterior horns of the lateral ventricles (in the peritrigonal region) ● White matter around the interventricular foramen of Monro.

Imaging Signs

▶ **Modality of choice**
MRI.

▶ **MRI and CT findings**
Hyperintensities on T2-weighted MR image, proton density, and FLAIR images ● Hypodensities (CT) in the white matter around the posterior horns of the lateral ventricles (peritrigonal region) and in the white matter around the interventricular foramen of Monro ● Ventricular enlargement with irregular contour, especially of the cella media and trigone of the lateral ventricles (incorporated cystic defects) ● Reduction of the periventricular white matter especially around the trigone of the lateral ventricles ● In severe cases, findings occur in the entire centrum semiovale ● Prominent sulci and a slender corpus callosum (truncus and splenium) are the result of degeneration of transcallosal fibers.

Clinical Aspects

▶ **Typical presentation/Course and prognosis**
Depending on severity, retarded development ● Subnormal intelligence ● Cerebral palsy.

▶ **Treatment options**
None.

▶ **What does the clinician want to know?**
Differentiate from other white-matter disease.

Congenital Malformations

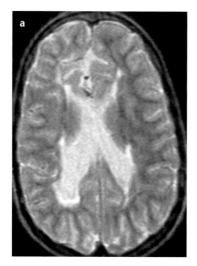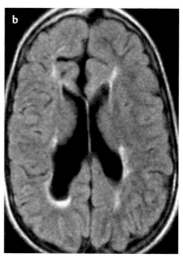

Fig. 11.9 a, b   Periventricular leukomalacia. Axial T2-weighted MR image (**a**) and axial FLAIR image (**b**). Bilateral focal hyperintensities in the subependymal white matter around the posterior and anterior horns of the lateral ventricles on T2-weighted images. The contour of the ventricle is partially irregular as a result of the incorporation of cystic defects.

Differential Diagnosis

Delayed myelination	– Thin band of normal white matter between the ventricle and unmyelinated white matter – Normal volume of white matter
Ventriculitis, meningitis	– Subependymal enhancement
Parasagittal medullary damage in term newborns	– Lesions in the parasagittal medulla and not in the subependymal region – No incorporation into the ventricles – Gliosis invariably present
Multiple sclerosis	– Often involves the corpus callosum and infratentorial structures – Lesions often oval – CSF findings

Tips and Pitfalls

Failing to obtain FLAIR images.

Selected References

Rezaie P et al. Periventricular leukomalacia, inflammation and white matter lesions within the developing nervous system. Neuropathology 2002; 22 (3): 106–132

Definition

▶ **Epidemiology**
   Frequency: 1:2300 (most common neurocutaneous syndrome).
▶ **Etiology, pathophysiology, pathogenesis**
   Autosomal dominant inheritance ● Gene locus on chromosome 17 (17q11) ● In 60% of cases the cause is a new mutation ● Form of secondary neurulation disturbance (defective neuronal proliferation, differentiation, and histogenesis) during the second through fourth months of pregnancy.
   Histology: Neurofibromas consist of Schwann cells, neurons, and collagen in an unorganized intercellular matrix ● In contrast to neurinomas (schwannomas) they have no capsule and have a higher content of collagen and elastin.
   Extracerebral manifestations: Plexiform neurofibromas of the head and neck ● Spinal neurofibromas.

Imaging Signs

▶ **Modality of choice**
   MRI.
▶ **CT findings**
   Dysplasia of the wing of the sphenoid ● Dysplasia of the bone along the lambdoid suture ● Calvarial defects.
▶ **MRI findings**
   Gliomas: Gliomas of the anterior visual pathway: Bilateral thickening of the optic nerve (optic chiasm, optic tract) without or with only minimal enhancement ● Gliomas of the tectum: thickening of the tectum and complete obliteration of the cerebral aqueduct with obstructive hydrocephalus ● Gliomas can also occur in the brainstem, cerebellum, and cerebral hemispheres.
   Myelin vacuolization: Hyperintensities on T2-weighted images in the brainstem, internal capsule, and basal ganglia as well as in the splenium of the corpus callosum and white matter of the cerebellum ● No enhancement after contrast administration ● Typically occurs only after age 3 years ● Number and size of lesions increase until age 10–12 years ● Myelin vacuolization is almost invariably absent in patients aged above 20 years ● Hyperintensity on non-contrast-enhanced T1-weighted images (reparative processes) ● Neurofibromas of the skull base and face are hyperintense to skeletal muscle on T1-weighted and T2-weighted images ● Lesions may enhance ● In dysplasia of the sphenoid wing, the temporal lobe herniates into the orbits.
▶ **DSA findings**
   Cerebral aneurysms ● Other vascular malformations.

Fig. 11.10 Neurofibromatosis type I. Axial T2-weighted MR image. Multiple bilateral hyperintensities in the internal capsule (myelin vacuolization; arrows).

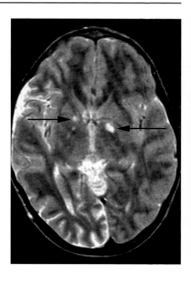

Clinical Aspects

▶ **Typical presentation/Course and prognosis**

Café-au-lait spots ● Cutaneous neurofibromas ● Protrusion of the globe, which may be caused by glioma of the optic nerve ● Occasionally pulsating exophthalmos ● Neuropsychologic deficits of varying severity ● Occasionally macrocephaly.
Diagnostic criteria:
 – At least five café-au-lait spots larger than 5 mm.
 – One plexiform neurofibroma or two or more cutaneous/subcutaneous neurofibromas.
 – Freckling in the axillary or inguinal region.
 – Dysplasia of the wing of the sphenoid or dysplasia of long bones.
 – Unilateral or bilateral gliomas of the optic nerve.
 – Two or more Lisch nodules (iris hamartomas).
 – Positive family history.

▶ **Treatment options**

Treatment of hydrocephalus ● Removal of neurofibromas or gliomas where indicated (gliomas of the optic nerve are removed only after confirming decrease in visual acuity or infiltrative growth) ● Surgical repair of sphenoid wing defect.

▶ **What does the clinician want to know?**

Depending on therapeutic relevance, follow-up of gliomas or hydrocephalus ● Demonstrate neurofibromas.

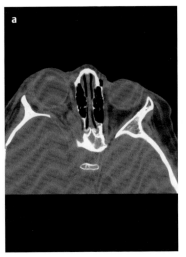 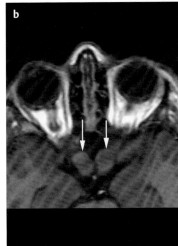

Fig. 11.11 a, b Axial CT of the orbits (**a**) and axial T1-weighted MR image (**b**). Hypoplasia of the greater and lesser wings of the right sphenoid with exophthalmos of the right eye (**a**). Bilateral gliomas of the optic nerve (**b**; arrows).

Differential Diagnosis

Benign stenosis of the *cerebral aqueduct*	– Proximal cerebral aqueduct dilated – Tectum of the midbrain thinned and superiorly displaced

Tips and Pitfalls

Misinterpreting the myelin vacuolization as a glioma.

Selected References

Aoki S et al. Neurofibromatosis types 1 and 2: cranial MR findings. Radiology 1989; 172 (2): 527–534

Griffiths PD. Sturge-Weber syndrome revisited: the role of neuroradiology. Neuropediatrics 1996; 27 (6): 284–294

Menor F et al. Neurofibromatosis type 1 in children: MR imaging and follow-up studies of central nervous system findings. Eur J Radiol 1998; 26 (2): 121–131

Definition

▶ **Epidemiology**
Frequency: 1:40 000.
▶ **Etiology, pathophysiology, pathogenesis**
Secondary neurulation disturbance (defective neuronal proliferation, differentiation, and histogenesis) during the second through fourth months of pregnancy ● Autosomal dominant inheritance ● Gene locus on chromosome 22.
Extracerebral manifestations: Multiple paraspinal schwannomas ● Spinal meningiomas and ependymomas.

Imaging Signs

▶ **Modality of choice**
MRI.
▶ **CT findings**
CT does not provide much useful information ● Inner auditory canal may be dilated.
▶ **MRI findings**
Neurinomas (schwannomas) of the vestibulocochlear nerve and other cranial nerves ● Multiple meningiomas.

Clinical Aspects

▶ **Typical presentation/Course and prognosis**
Balance impairments and tinnitus without characteristic skin findings ● Posterior subcapsular cataract is an early symptom ● Peak age of manifestation of acoustic neurinomas is 10–20 years.
Diagnostic criteria: The presence of two of the following three clinical criteria is diagnostic:
– Bilateral tumors of the eighth cranial nerve.
– Patient is an immediate relative of a patient with neurofibromatosis type II and has either a unilateral tumor of the eighth cranial nerve or two of the following manifestations: neurofibroma, meningioma, glioma, neurinoma, posterior subcapsular cataract, or cerebral calcification.
– Either a unilateral acoustic neurinoma and multiple meningiomas or one of these two manifestations in combination with neurofibroma, meningioma, glioma, neurinoma, posterior subcapsular cataract, or cerebral calcification.
▶ **Treatment options**
Removal of the neurinomas or meningiomas where indicated.
▶ **What does the clinician want to know?**
Follow-up of the neurinomas or meningiomas.

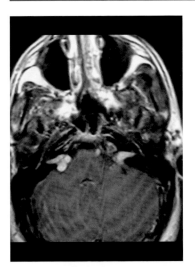

Fig. 11.12   Neurofibromatosis type II. Bilateral acoustic neurinomas. Axial T1-weighted MR image after contrast administration.

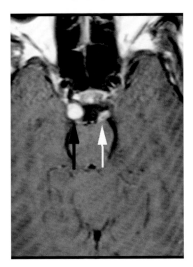

Fig. 11.13   Left oculomotor neurinoma (white arrow) and right clinoid process meningioma (black arrow). Axial T1-weighted MR image after contrast administration (patient from Fig. 11.**12**).

Fig. 11.14   Left frontal meningioma (arrow). Axial T1-weighted MR image after contrast administration (patient from Fig. 11.**12**).

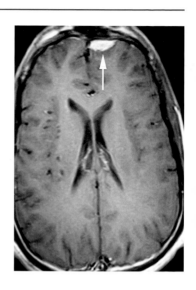

Differential Diagnosis

Schwannomas without neurofibromatosis type II   – Usually unilateral

Tips and Pitfalls

Misinterpreting as neurofibromatosis type I.

Selected References

Aoki S et al. Neurofibromatosis types 1 and 2: cranial MR findings. Radiology 1989; 172 (2): 527–534

Herron J et al. Intra-cranial manifestations of the neurocutaneous syndromes. Clin Radiol 2000; 55 (2): 82–98

Definition

▶ **Epidemiology**
Incidence: 1:10 000–1:50 000 per year ● Second most common neurocutaneous disorder.

▶ **Etiology, pathophysiology, pathogenesis**
Secondary neurulation disturbance (defective neuronal proliferation, differentiation, and histogenesis) during the second through fourth months of pregnancy ● Autosomal dominant inheritance ● Two gene loci have been described to date: 9q34 and 16p13.

Imaging Signs

▶ **Modality of choice**
MRI.

▶ **CT findings**
Images demonstrate calcified tubers or calcified subependymal hamartomas.

▶ **MRI findings**
Cortical tubers: Usually multiple ● Most commonly occur in the supratentorial region ● In newborns, they are hyperintense to the adjacent yet unmyelinated white matter on T1-weighted images and hypointense on T2-weighted images ● In older children, the center of the tubers is hypointense to white matter on T1-weighted images and hyperintense on T2-weighted images ● In the mature brain lesions, may be isointense on T1-weighted images but are practically invariably hyperintense on T2-weighted images ● Calcification may occur ● FLAIR and magnetization transfer provide more diagnostic information with respect to the size and number of lesions.
Subependymal hamartomas: Subependymal nodules are most commonly found along the ventricular contour of the caudate nucleus immediately posterior to the interventricular foramen of Monro, but also at other sites ● In newborns, lesions are hyperintense relative to the adjacent, yet unmyelinated white matter on T1-weighted images and hypointense on T2-weighted images ● As the brain matures, lesions increasingly appear isointense to white matter on T1-weighted and T2-weighted images ● Nodules calcify, but not before the end of the first year of life ● Enhancement may occur but is of no clinical significance.
Subependymal giant cell astrocytomas: Usually lie near the interventricular foramen of Monro ● Usually larger than 12 mm ● Often lead to obstructive hydrocephalus ● Invariably enhance ● May calcify.
White-matter lesions: Signal pattern is identical to that of cortical tubers ● FLAIR and magnetization transfer provides more diagnostic information.

Clinical Aspects

▶ **Typical presentation/Course and prognosis**
"White spots" of melanin hypopigmentation ● Facial angiofibromas: reddish nodules, initially the size of a grain of rice, later larger butterfly-shaped lesions

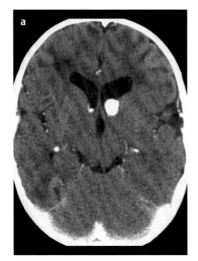 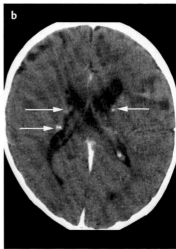

Fig. 11.15 a, b Tuberous sclerosis. Axial CT after contrast administration. Calcified subependymal tumor in the anterior horn of the left lateral ventricle (giant cell astrocytoma, **a**). Multiple enhancing subependymal nodules, some calcified (hamartomas), along the walls of the lateral ventricle (**b**; arrows). Multiple cortical and subcortical tubers on both sides in the frontal temporooccipital and occipital regions (hamartia; **a, b**).

on the cheeks, nasolabial folds, and nose ● Shagreen patches: cutaneous lesions of variable size with leathery proliferations of connective tissue that have a predilection for the lumbosacral region ● Generalized seizures.

▶ **Treatment options**
Symptomatic treatment of the seizures ● CSF drainage in hydrocephalus.

▶ **What does the clinician want to know?**
Associated malformations? ● Hydrocephalus?

Differential Diagnosis

Viral and other encephalitides with calcifications in the vicinity of the ventricles (rubella, cytomegalovirus infection, toxoplasmosis)	– Other signs of tuberous sclerosis are absent

Selected References

Crino PB et al. New developments in the neurobiology of the tuberous sclerosis complex. Neurology 1999; 53 (7): 1384–1390

Evans JC et al. The radiological appearances of tuberous sclerosis. Br J Radiol 2000; 73 (865): 91–98

Sparagana SP et al. Tuberous sclerosis complex. Curr Opin Neurol 2000; 13 (2): 115–119

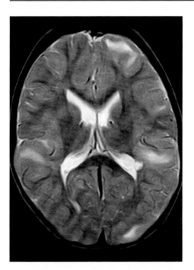

Fig. 11.16 Tuberous sclerosis. Axial T2-weighted MR image. Multiple tubers with high signal intensity on T2-weighted images. Subependymal nodule at the trigone of the left lateral ventricle with high signal intensity.

Congenital Malformations

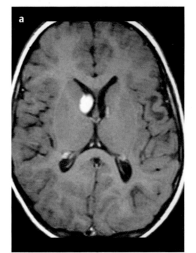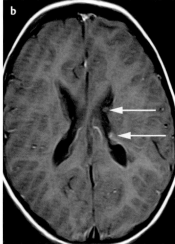

Fig. 11.17 a, b Tuberous sclerosis. Axial T1-weighted MR images after contrast administration. Enhancing subependymal tumor in the anterior horn of the right lateral ventricle in the vicinity of the interventricular foramen of Monro (subependymal giant cell astrocytoma). Enhancing subependymal hamartomas (**b**; arrows).

Definition

▶ **Epidemiology**
Fourth most common neurocutaneous syndrome.

▶ **Etiology, pathophysiology, pathogenesis**
Secondary neurulation disturbance (defective neuronal proliferation, differentiation, and histogenesis) during the second through fourth months of pregnancy • No sex or racial predilection.

Imaging Signs

▶ **Modality of choice**
MRI and CT.

▶ **CT findings**
Cortical calcifications • Loss of brain volume.

▶ **MRI findings**
Broad thickening of the pia mater with pronounced enhancement on T1-weighted images consistent with meningeal angioma • Volume loss in the affected hemisphere with shift of midline structures • Calvarial thickening • Asymmetry of the skull with enlargement of the ipsilateral frontal sinus • Increased enhancement in the choroid plexus on the same side as the pial angioma • In 10–30% of cases, congenital glaucoma with buphthalmos is present.

Clinical Aspects

▶ **Typical presentation/Course and prognosis**
Congenital facial port wine stain (nevus flammeus) follows the course of the first branch of the trigeminal nerve • In 5–10% of cases, a nevus can also be demonstrated in other regions of the body • Epilepsy (complex partial seizures) • There may be hemiplegia contralateral to the facial nevus.

▶ **Treatment options**
Symptomatic treatment of the epilepsy.

▶ **What does the clinician want to know?**
Severity of the hemiatrophy.

Tips and Pitfalls

Confusing this disease with other less common phakomatoses such as Wyburn–Mason syndrome, Klippel–Trenaunay–Weber syndrome, or meningioangiomatosis.

Selected References

Griffiths PD. Sturge–Weber syndrome revisited: the role of neuroradiology. Neuropediatrics 1996; 27 (6): 284–294

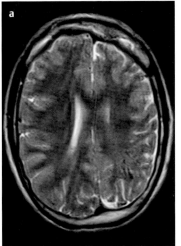
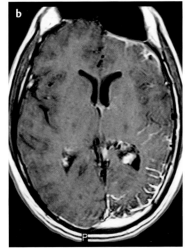

Fig. 11.18 a, b   Sturge–Weber syndrome. Axial T2-weighted MR image (**a**) and axial T1-weighted MR image after contrast administration (**b**). Significant volume loss in the left cerebral hemisphere (**a, b**). Reduced signal intensities in the parietooccipital region in the cortical band on T2-weighted images (**a**) consistent with cortical calcifications. Abnormally increased enhancement on the surface of the brain in the left parietooccipital region consistent with a typical pial angioma (**b**).

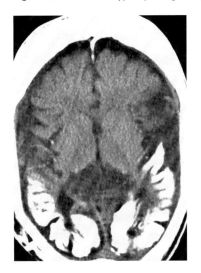

Fig. 11.19   Axial CT. Typical bilateral bands of cortical calcifications in the parietooccipital regions. Loss of brain volume is most pronounced in the parietooccipital region.

Definition
....

▶ **Epidemiology**
Incidence: 1:36 000.
▶ **Etiology, pathophysiology, pathogenesis**
Form of secondary neurulation disturbance (defective neuronal proliferation, differentiation, and histogenesis) during the second through fourth months of pregnancy • Autosomal dominant inheritance • Gene defect on chromosome 3p25–26 • The disease receives its name from angiomatosis retinae (von Hippel) and hemangioblastoma (see p. 172) of the cerebellum (Lindau tumor).
Extracerebral manifestations: Spinal hemangioblastomas • Renal and pancreatic cysts • Renal carcinoma • Pheochromocytoma or cystadenoma of the epididymis • Unlike in neurofibromatosis, Sturge–Weber syndrome, and tuberous sclerosis, there are typical skin findings.

Imaging Signs
....

▶ **Modality of choice**
MRI.
▶ **CT findings**
Cerebellar hemangioblastomas: Hypodense cerebellar mass with enhancing tumor nodules.
Papillary cystadenomas of endolymphatic sac: Mass on the posterior surface of the petrous bone at the vestibular aqueduct • Bone destruction • Central calcification.
▶ **MRI findings**
Cerebellar hemangioblastomas: Fluid-filled cyst with small, strongly enhancing vascularized tumor nodules • Solid lesions are present in 30% of cases • Rarely, cysts will not enhance at all • Often there are flow voids (usually tubular) on proton density and T2-weighted images • Spontaneous hemorrhage occasionally occurs.
Papillary cystadenomas of endolymphatic sac: Enhancing mass with an inhomogeneous MR signal on the posterior surface of the petrous bone at the vestibular aqueduct.
▶ **DSA findings**
Densely opacified tangle of vessels in the early arterial phase (see p. 174).

Clinical Aspects
....

▶ **Typical presentation/Course and prognosis**
Central retinal angioma leads to loss of visual acuity • Cerebellar signs • Back pain • Elevated intracranial pressure • Regular screening for renal cell carcinoma and pheochromocytoma is indicated.
▶ **Treatment options**
Surgical removal of larger hemangioblastomas.

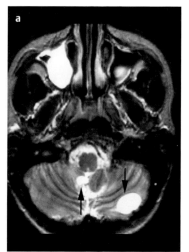

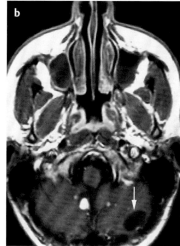

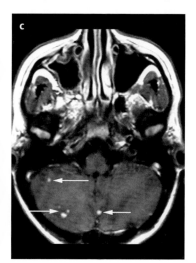

Fig. 11.20 a–c Von Hippel–Lindau syndrome. Axial T2-weighted MR image (**a**) and axial T1-weighted MR images after contrast administration (**b,c**). Multiple tumors, some cystic (**a**), in both cerebellar hemispheres with strong nodular enhancement (**b,c**; arrows).

▶ **What does the clinician want to know?**
Number, location, and size of the hemangioblastomas ● Spinal hemangioblastomas?

Differential Diagnosis
....

Hemangioblastomas without	– Usually solitary
von Hippel–Lindau syndrome	– No central retinal angioma

Selected References

Torreggiani WC et al. Von Hippel–Lindau disease: a radiological essay. Clin Radiol 2002; 57 (8): 670–680

Definition

▶ **Etiology, pathophysiology, pathogenesis**
Form of secondary neurulation disturbance (defective ventral induction) in the fifth to tenth weeks of pregnancy • Defective differentiation and division of the prosencephalon at the end of the fifth week of pregnancy • No sex predilection • Associated with trisomy 13, trisomy 18, facial dysmorphias such as hypertelorism.
Three forms: Alobar, semilobar, and lobar holoprosencephaly.

Imaging Signs

▶ **Modality of choice**
MRI • CT is also suitable in alobar and semilobar holoprosencephaly.
▶ **CT and MRI findings**
Alobar holoprosencephaly: Thalami are fused • Third ventricle, longitudinal fissure, falx cerebri, and corpus callosum are absent • Cerebrum adheres to the rostral portion of the skull cavity • Single large ventricle communicating with a large posterior cyst • Orbits may also be fused • Azygos anterior cerebral artery.
Semilobar holoprosencephaly: Longitudinal fissure • Posterior rudiments of the falx cerebri are present • Frontal brain is underdeveloped and fused • Thalami are partially separated • Rudimentary temporal horns of the lateral ventricles • Incomplete hippocampus • Septum pellucidum is absent • Truncus of the corpus callosum is absent; splenium is present.
Lobar holoprosencephaly: CT provides little useful information • Frontal horns of the lateral ventricles are hypoplastic • Posterior half of the corpus callosum is present • Longitudinal fissure and falx cerebri are present and extend into the frontal portion of the brain • Anterior falx cerebri is occasionally hypoplastic.

Clinical Aspects

▶ **Typical presentation/Course and prognosis**
Alobar holoprosencephaly: Usually stillborn or surviving for only a very short time.
Lobar holoprosencephaly: Slightly or only moderately retarded development • Hypothalamic and pituitary hypofunction • Impaired vision.
▶ **Treatment options**
Symptomatic treatment of hypothalamic and pituitary hypofunction.
▶ **What does the clinician want to know?**
Differentiation of the various forms.

Differential Diagnosis

Dysgenesis of the corpus callosum with colpocephaly	– Posterior portions of the corpus callosum are absent, not the anterior portions

Fig. 11.21 Alobar holoprosencephaly. Axial T1-weighted MR image. Single large ventricle with "pancake" cerebrum in the rostral portion of the skull cavity.

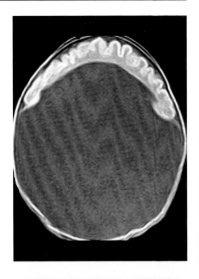

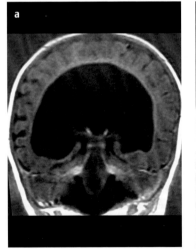

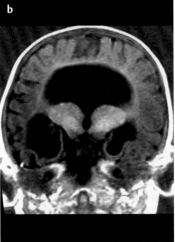

Fig. 11.22 a, b Semilobar holoprosencephaly. Coronal T1-weighted MR images. Rudimentary temporal horns of the lateral ventricles, incomplete hippocampus, partially separated thalami, absent septum pellucidum.

Tips and Pitfalls

Misinterpreting as hydrocephalus or colpocephaly with dysgenesis of the corpus callosum.

Selected References

Barkovich AJ. Magnetic resonance imaging: role in the understanding of cerebral malformations. Brain Dev 2002; 24 (1): 2–12

Fig. 12.1 Axial T1-weighted gradient echo MR image. Sharply demarcated hypointense halo around the orbital muscles at the boundary with the orbital fat (water–fat interface).

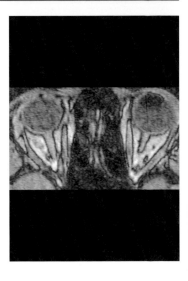

Chemical Shift Artifact

▶ **Cause**

The slight difference in the resonance frequency of protons in different tissues (fat, muscle) simulates a difference in spatial encoding, leading to spatial misregistration (first-order chemical shift artifact). In gradient echo sequences, the lack of the 180° rephasing pulse in certain echo times (TE) means that water and fat signals cancel each other out due to their opposed phases (second-order chemical shift artifact).

▶ **Remedy**

Increasing receiver bandwidth (this applies only to the first-order chemical shift artifact); in a second-order artifact, echo time must be adjusted according to the field strength so as to avoid opposed-phase imaging of fat and water.

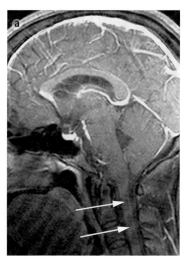 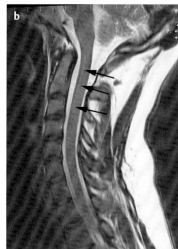

Fig. 12.2 a, b Sagittal T1-weighted MR image (**a**) and sagittal T2-weighted MR image (**b**). T1-weighted images show a longitudinal hypointensity (**a**; arrows) and T2-weighted images a corresponding hyperintensity (**b**; arrows) along the spinal cord, simulating a syrinx.

Truncation Artifact (Gibbs Artifact)

▶ **Cause**

Result of the Fourier transformation in image reconstruction. Theoretically the MR signal represents an infinite summation of sine waves of various frequencies, phases, and amplitudes, whereas in practice the number of frequencies is finite. This causes overshooting or undershooting in tissue interfaces with high contrast, resulting in heightened demarcation, apparent widening, or displacement of the edges.

▶ **Remedy**

Increasing the number of phase-encoding steps, reducing the size of the scanning field, increasing the matrix.

Fig. 12.3 Axial T1-weighted MR image. Signal void with hyperintense ring.

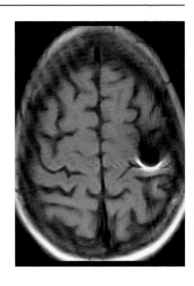

Susceptibility Artifact

▶ **Cause**

Occurs along the boundaries of substances of different magnetic susceptibility. This produces a localized disturbance of the magnetic field (air–bone, metal, calcific deposits).

▶ **Remedy**

Decreasing the echo time, using spin echo sequences where possible, using lower field strengths.

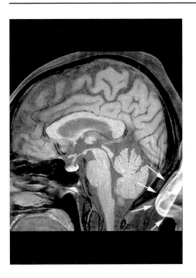

Fig. 12.4 Sagittal T1-weighted MR image. When the scanning field is too small, the patient's nose is visualized on the posterior part of the image (arrows).

Aliasing or Wrap Around

▶ **Cause**

This occurs when the scanning field is smaller than the size of the object in the phase-encoding direction or (in 3D sequences) in the slice direction. Because the phase-encoding steps are only defined in a range from 0 to 360°, a phase shift of 364° will be assigned to the spatial position 4° for example. More precisely, the range is from − 180° to + 180°. Thus, + 184 = − 176.

▶ **Remedy**

Expanding the scanning field in the phase-encoding direction, oversampling in the phase-encoding direction (i.e., more phase-encoding steps are recorded than are required for image reconstruction).

Ghosting

▶ **Cause**

Occurs due to nonpulsatile or pulsatile flow of blood or CSF or other periodic motions. Occur in the phase-encoding direction. The severity of these artifacts increases with the signal intensity of the moving tissue and with the speed of motion. Nonperiodic motion produces image noise in the phase-encoding direction. The distances between the individual artifacts depend on the primary direction of motion, the amplitude of motion, and the periodicity: the faster the motion, the larger the distances.

Flow artifacts are classified in various orders.

▶ **Remedy**

Eliminating the motion (immobilizing the head), suppressing the signal of the moving tissue with saturation pulses, pulse triggering, changing the phase-encoding direction (this usually does not change the artifact but often ensures that it will not occur in the region of interest).

The most important remedy with respect to choice of sequence is gradient moment nulling, flow compensation by means of special gradient settings.

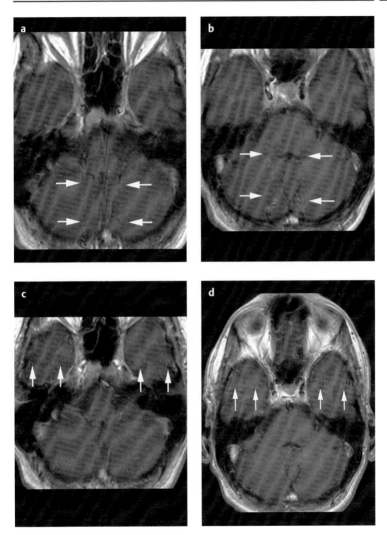

Fig. 12.5 a–d Axial T1-weighted MR images after contrast administration. Phase-encoding directions are anterior-posterior in **a** and **b** and lateral in **c** and **d**. Pulsation of the internal carotid artery produces longitudinal artifacts (arrows; **a, b**) or transverse artifacts (arrows; **c, d**), depending on the phase-encoding direction.

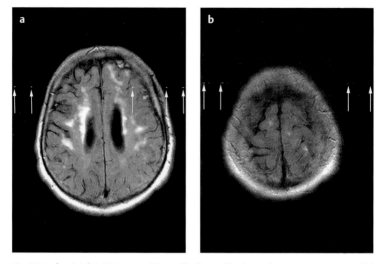

Fig. 12.6 a, b Axial FLAIR images. Zipper-like lines of high signal intensity appear parallel to the phase-encoding direction (arrows).

Zipper Artifact

► **Cause**

Occurs as a result of a "receiver leak" such as from an exogenous high-frequency source when the doors of the scanner room are not completely closed or from an insufficiently shielded pulse oximeter in the scanner room.

The artifact is manifested in the phase-encoding direction with high-frequency interference sources (leak or electronic device), and in the direction of frequency encoding with low-frequency interference sources (such as a defective "buzzing" light bulb in the scanner room).

► **Remedy**

Eliminating the leak and moving equipment outside the scanner room wherever possible. Do not feed electrical cables through access openings in the wall (they emit interference frequencies).

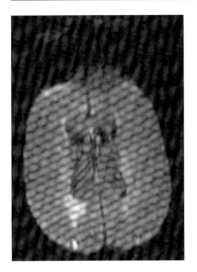

Fig. 12.7 Axial T1-weighted MR image. A fine checkerboard pattern homogeneously covers the entire image.

Point Artifact

▶ **Cause**

Insufficient humidity in scanner room. This results in spontaneous discharges that create a visual image. ● Defective cables. ● Faults in the high-frequency amplifier unit.

▶ **Remedy**

Increase humidity. ● Call engineer.

Selected References

Elster AD et al.: Questions and Answers in Magnetic Resonance Imaging. St. Louis: Mosby, 2001

Tsuchihashi T. [Artifact of MRI]. Nippon Hoshasen Gijutsu Gakkai Zasshi 2003; 59 (11): 1370–1377

Fig. 13.1 Axial CT, bone window. Status post surgery for aneurysm of the right internal carotid artery, showing metal clip.

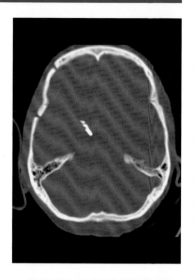

Fig. 13.2 Axial CT, bone window. Coil (arrow) in the middle meningeal artery placed after endovascular devascularization of a meningioma.

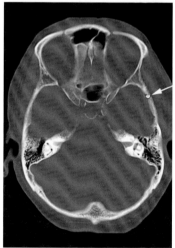

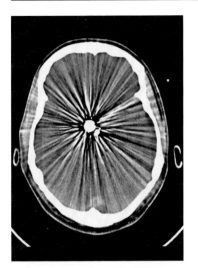

Fig. 13.3 Axial CT, soft-tissue window. Endovascular occlusion of an aneurysm of the internal carotid artery. Coil artifacts.

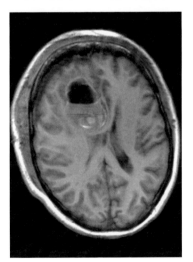

Fig. 13.4 Axial noncontrasted T1-weighted MR image. Postoperative parenchymal defect following resection of a right frontal brain tumor. Two interfaces are visible in the defect. There is an anterior boundary between seroma and air and a posterior boundary between seroma and blood.

Fig. 13.5 Axial T1-weighted MR image after contrast administration. Postoperative parenchymal defect following resection of a left frontal glioma. The tumor has been removed, and slight reactive enhancement is visible along the margins of the defect.

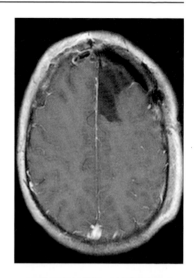

Fig. 13.6 Coronal T1-weighted MR image after contrast administration. A subdural hematoma has occurred postoperatively. The meningeal enhancement is reactive.

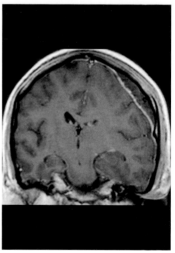

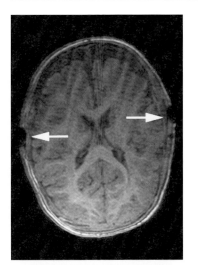

Fig. 13.7 Axial T1-weighted MR image. MRI after surgery to correct a trigonocephalic malformation. Bilateral temporal metal artifacts from implants.

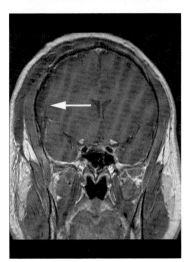

Fig. 13.8 Coronal T1-weighted MR image after contrast administration. Bone cover of Palacos bone cement in the right temporoparietal region (arrow).

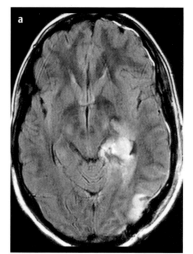 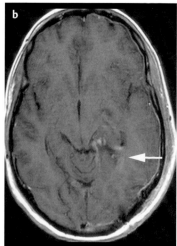

Fig. 13.9 a, b Axial FLAIR image (**a**) and T1-weighted MR image after contrast administration (**b**). Following subtotal resection of a left temporal glioma, portions of the tumor
remain in the hippocampus and occipital region. The mass is detectable on the FLAIR
image because of its increased signal. There is also enhancement at the margin of the
residual tumor (arrow, **b**), a sign of a compromised blood-brain barrier.

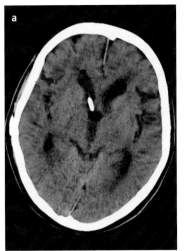
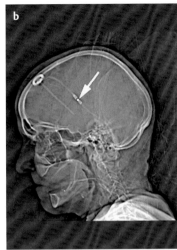

Fig. 13.10 a, b Axial CT, soft-tissue window (**a**) and lateral plain skull radiograph (**b**). Hydrocephalus following surgical shunt procedure. The tip of the shunt catheter is projected on the anterior horn of the right lateral ventricle. A small air inclusion is also visualized in the anterior horn of the ventricle. The plain skull radiograph shows the course of the shunt system with adjustable valve (**b**; arrow).